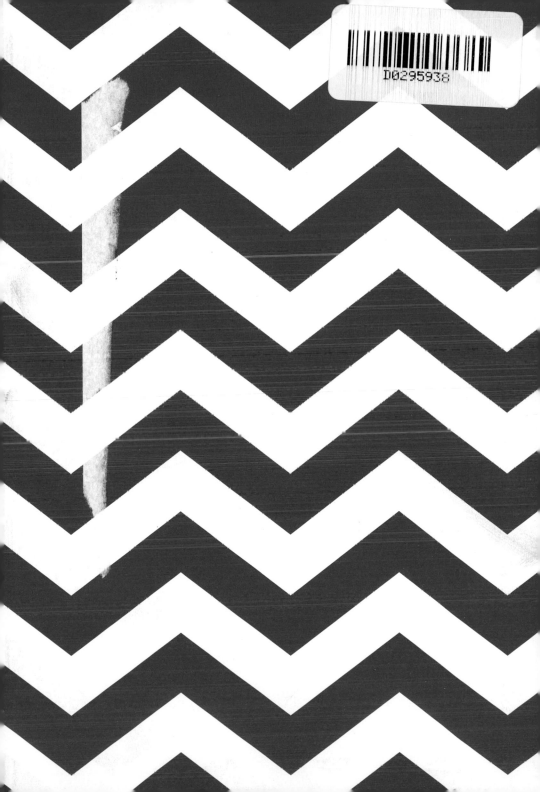

NEW MUM, YOU'RE DOING BRILLIANTLY

What do new mums want most of all (apart from sleep)? They want someone to tell them what they're feeling is 'normal'. That they're doing ok. That *they* will be ok.

The New Mum's Notebook, written by Amy Ransom – mum of three and creator of the Surviving Motherhood blog – does all this and more.

From night feeds, napping and weaning, to which films to cue up on Netflix, finding some headspace and getting all the support, coffee and cake you need, Amy has been there – and this is the book she wishes she'd had by her side.

Divided into the first 12 months of motherhood, with 304 pages of reassurance, love and humour, as well as spaces to scribble thoughts, feelings and memories from those crazy early days, *The New Mum's Notebook* will nurture a new mum in *however* she chooses to raise her baby. Whether it's her first or her fifth.

Word on the street is it's *almost* worth having another baby for.

GET IN TOUCH

Share and tag your photos of
The New Mum's Notebook #TheNewMumsNotebook

Visit the Surviving Motherhood blog
www.amyransom.com
Facebook.com/amyransomwrites
Instagram.com/survivingmotherhood_
Twitter.com/amyransom_

Sign up for support and inspiration at
www.thenewmumsnotebook.co.uk

THE NEW MUM'S NOTEBOOK

A sanity-saving journal for all new mums

Amy Ransom

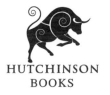

HUTCHINSON
BOOKS

Hutchinson
20 Vauxhall Bridge Road
London SW1V 2SA

Hutchinson is part of the Penguin Random House group of companies
whose addresses can be found at global.penguinrandomhouse.com

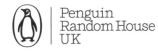

First published in the United Kingdom by Amy Ransom in 2016
First published by Hutchinson in 2017

www.penguin.co.uk

A CIP catalogue record for this book is available from the British Library.

ISBN 9781786331168

Printed and bound in Italy by L.E.G.O. S.p.A.

The information in this book has been compiled by way of general guidance
in relation to the specific subjects addressed. It is not a substitute for and
is not to be relied on for medical, healthcare, pharmaceutical or other
professional advice. Please consult your GP before changing, stopping or
starting any medical treatment. Neither the author nor the publisher shall
be liable or responsible for any loss or damage allegedly arising from any
information or suggestion in this book.

So far as the author is aware, the information given is correct and up to date
as at the time of publication. Neither the publisher nor the author assumes any
responsibility for errors or changes that occur after publication.

Penguin Random House is committed to a sustainable future for our business,
our readers and our planet. This book is made from Forest Stewardship Council®
certified paper.

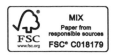

For Eva, Ivy and Joseph.
Always 'in my heart'.

And for every new mum out there who doubts herself.
You're going to be ok.

Contents

Dear New Mum,

Congratulations on your teeny tiny bundle. You grew a human! That officially makes you awesome. How are you feeling, now the dust has settled a bit? Probably a mixture of happy, knackered, confused and anxious. Because it's weird isn't it, becoming a mum? Pretty over-whelming, I'd say. I remember those early weeks so well. That feeling of exhaustion at the end of the day and thinking, 'Do I really have to do all this again tomorrow?'

Everything feels so permanent when you're a new mum. You think you'll never sleep again. How on earth do you even get a baby to go to sleep? Without rocking them? To stay asleep? And you daren't put the baby down. Ever. In case they detonate everything in their path.

But you will sleep again. As your baby grows, they'll become more satisfied and wake less for milk. You'll find ways to comfort them and settle them for sleep. Maybe you'll rock them. Maybe they'll self-soothe. It doesn't really matter right now. Because it only takes three days to break a habit. So if you do create habits you want to change later, you'll be able to. In three days. When you're ready. When you're strong enough. When it matters.

And it really does get easier. I promise you. Everything changes. Constantly. Remember, 'This too shall pass'. Phases come and go and you will learn to weather the storms. To be that palm tree that survives a tsunami because it bends with the wind. Mums have strength and resources unlike anyone else.

Whenever you can, go with the flow because your baby will keep you on your toes. They'll sleep. Then suddenly they'll have a couple of days when sleep's the last thing on their mind. Because they're teething. Or having a growth spurt. Or just don't feel like it. Likewise with food, one day they'll eat sweet potato. The next? They'll be flinging it across the room in disgust. And protesting with a hunger strike. It will make you feel anxious. Out of control. Tearful. Try to go with it and you'll feel more relaxed.

You're probably discovering that alongside 'challenging' and 'tiring', motherhood can be monotonous. Sometimes lonely. So get yourself out every day. For a walk in the park. Feel the sun on your head. Meet a friend for coffee. Or make the most of the fact that your baby can't move yet and do some good-fashioned retail therapy.

Never agonise over the decisions you make. None of us get it right all of the time. We can only do what we think is best. Stand proud in all of your decisions. You don't have to justify yourself to anyone. Ever. Your baby. Your rules. Try not to waste time feeling guilty. It starts the minute you give birth and will take over your soul if you let it. Remember, you're doing your best and it IS good enough.

It's ok to have undesirable thoughts. You don't have to love every second of every day. I remember once saying, 'If she doesn't sleep soon, I'm going to fling her out of the window.' I had no intention of doing it. But I needed to vent my frustration. And say something angry. To convey just how tired I was. You are not a bad mother for thinking thoughts like this. You're a very normal one.

Don't worry about the state of your relationship. Having a baby will challenge you both in different ways. You'll feel knackered and want to strangle your partner when they say insensitive things like, 'I'm exhausted.' They'll be feeling helpless because their experience of parenthood isn't quite the same as yours. They didn't grow your baby or give birth. So save yourself the anguish, ask them to hug you instead and save the moaning for your mum friends. Who will completely and utterly get everything you're feeling. Before you've even said it.

Finally. Be kind to yourself. Every day. Embrace the fourth trimester. Always remember that moments pass. Talk to other mums. Accept any offers of help. And put your hand up if you're struggling. Because motherhood is the most challenging job most of us have ever done. And there are no prizes for flying solo. Once you open up, you'll be surprised by just how many mums are feeling exactly the way you are.

It DOES get easier. I promise. You're doing brilliantly.   Amy x

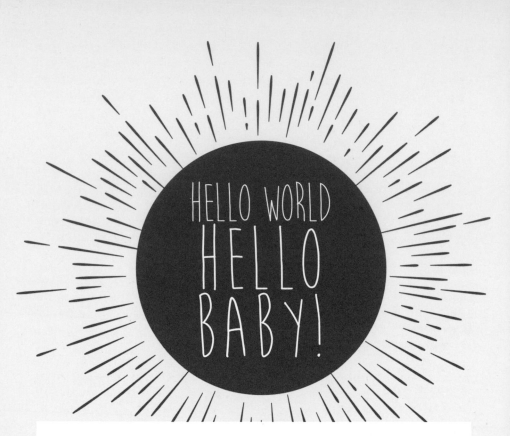

When and where you were born: ....

....

How teeny you were: ....

What we called you: ....

What we didn't call you: ....

What I want to remember about this day:

....

....

MONTH ONE

Welcome
to
Motherhood.

THE FIRST 12 DAYS WITH A NEWBORN
(WHAT YOU CAN EXPECT)

DAY ONE 'I CAN DO ANYTHING!'

There is NO day like this one. The one where you meet your baby. Regardless of how your baby arrived or how sore you are, you did it! This day will be spent marvelling at that teeny, tiny human being that YOU made. Eating toast. Sharing the arrival of your new addition. And feeling so relieved that both you and your baby are safe. You'll be on top of the world, despite the after pains and feeling completely knackered. This is how insanely euphoric day one really is.

DAY TWO 'WOW. MY BABY IS GOOD'

You've had the first night with your newborn, who may well have fooled you by sleeping five hours or more in one stretch. 'Wow. My baby is good,' you think. You're surprised how good you feel. Not yet tired enough to mind the night feeds, you actually enjoy having those little pink fingers gripping yours at 3.00AM in the morning. You'll possibly have some visitors. And the adoration from everyone around you will further enhance that post-labour glow you're sporting.

DAY THREE THE 'BOOB JOB' PHASE

Ugh. What's that pressure on your chest? You wake up and look down to find that, overnight, your body's been possessed. By a glamour model. And a dairy cow. Yes, whilst you were sleeping, your milk's come in. And the pain is excruciating. The only thing that relieves it is cold cabbage leaves from the freezer or, if you're breastfeeding, feeding your baby. But this in turn makes you feel like someone is poking hot pins through your nipples. At the same time, your happy hormones decide to take leave. Suddenly you feel low, tired and teary.

DAY FOUR TEARS AND MORE TEARS

The Baby Blues have probably well and truly hit. And although they're usually gone in a few days, whilst you've got them, it's hard to see beyond them. Expect to cry. A lot. Often for no reason at all.

It's perfectly normal. The departure of the post-labour endorphins, the dramatic hormonal changes and the discomfort of your milk coming in can make you feel irrational. Try not to think. Or to rationalise your feelings. Rest assured that this phase will pass. And rest.

DAY FIVE REALITY BITES. OUCH

You wake up feeling more like yourself. Albeit a tired and slightly more frazzled version. The tears have subsided. Leaving you feeling a bit numb. You're suddenly slightly overwhelmed that you have to do this *every* day. The night feeds have lost their appeal and you may have had THAT night. The one where your baby refuses to settle ALL night no matter what you do. The one where you cry because you're so tired. The one where you give your other half a kick in the back because they get to sleep while you don't. This night has a purpose. It moves you into your new reality.

DAYS SIX TO NINE GETTING ON WITH IT

This is a relatively peaceful phase. You've had the extreme initial emotions and now you're just doing it. If you're feeding, it's becoming a little more comfortable. You might even have won some small victories like getting the baby to settle in its cot. And your uterus is probably back where it started. Even if your belly button isn't.

DAY TEN 'ON YER BIKE'

If all is going well, the midwife will discharge you. If it's your first baby, you may do this baby business again. If it's your last baby, however, expect to feel a sudden wave of sadness and nostalgia. Because the thought that you will never do this again can do strange things to you, such as a) cling to your midwife's leg b) beg her never to leave you c) get pregnant.

DAYS ELEVEN-TWELVE WELCOME TO MOTHERHOOD

Motherhood doesn't end at day 12. You don't graduate, pass GO or collect £200. What does happen during this period is acceptance. Acceptance of your new life. The tiredness. The demands. The responsibility. At this point you start to realise that you can do this. Because you're already doing it.

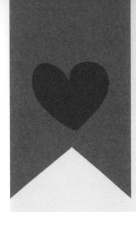

ON THIS DAY

DATE: _____

If it's all feeling a bit crazy, just know that it does get easier.

MY NOTES
(WHAT I LOVED, FELT, WISHED, NEEDED, STRUGGLED WITH, OVERCAME)

....

....

....

....

....

....

....

....

....

....

....

TO DO LIST

❏ ....

❏ ....

❏ ....

❏ ....

❏ ....

THINGS TO REMEMBER
(BECAUSE A BABY ATE MY BRAIN)

....

....

....

....

....

MEMORIES TO RECALL
(YEARS FROM NOW)

....

....

....

....

....

BABY NOTES
(WHAT YOU DID, LOVED, NEEDED)

....

....

....

....

....

....

....

....

....

....

....

....

FEEDING NOTES
(TIME, DURATION/AMOUNT)

....

....

....

....

....

....

....

....

....

....

....

....

BE KIND
TO YOURSELF.
EVERY DAY.
ALWAYS REMEMBER
THAT MOMENTS PASS.

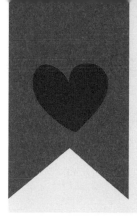

ON THIS DAY

DATE: _____

Drink water. Dehydration can cause headaches and blurred vision, especially if you're breastfeeding.

MY NOTES
(WHAT I LOVED, FELT, WISHED, NEEDED, STRUGGLED WITH, OVERCAME)

....

....

....

....

....

....

....

....

....

....

....

TO DO LIST

☐ ....

☐ ....

☐ ....

☐ ....

☐ ....

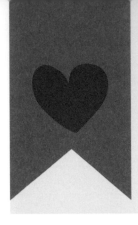

ON THIS DAY

DATE: _____

Enjoy cuddling your baby. There is nothing like the feeling of a newborn on your chest.

MY NOTES
(WHAT I LOVED, FELT, WISHED, NEEDED, STRUGGLED WITH, OVERCAME)

....

....

....

....

....

....

....

....

....

....

....

TO DO LIST

❏ ....

❏ ....

❏ ....

❏ ....

❏ ....

THINGS TO REMEMBER
(BECAUSE A BABY ATE MY BRAIN)

....

....

....

....

....

MEMORIES TO RECALL
(YEARS FROM NOW)

....

....

....

....

....

BABY NOTES
(WHAT YOU DID, LOVED, NEEDED)

....

....

....

....

....

....

....

....

....

....

....

....

....

FEEDING NOTES
(TIME, DURATION/AMOUNT)

....

....

....

....

....

....

....

....

....

....

....

....

....

TODAY I WAS AMAZING.

DATE: ....

BECAUSE: ....

....

....

....

....

....

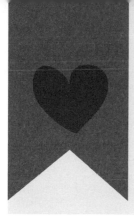

ON THIS DAY

DATE: _____

Don't fill your time rushing around after visitors. The early weeks are for rest and recovery.

MY NOTES
(WHAT I LOVED, FELT, WISHED, NEEDED, STRUGGLED WITH, OVERCAME)

....

....

....

....

....

....

....

....

....

....

....

TO DO LIST

☐ ....

☐ ....

☐ ....

☐ ....

☐ ....

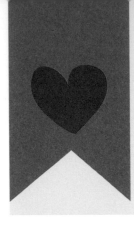

ON THIS DAY

DATE: _____

Going out for the first time on your own is scary. But fresh air is good for the soul. You can do this.

MY NOTES
(WHAT I LOVED, FELT, WISHED, NEEDED, STRUGGLED WITH, OVERCAME)

....

....

....

....

....

....

....

....

....

....

....

....

TO DO LIST

❑ ....

❑ ....

❑ ....

❑ ....

❑ ....

THINGS TO REMEMBER
(BECAUSE A BABY ATE MY BRAIN)

....

....

....

....

....

MEMORIES TO RECALL
(YEARS FROM NOW)

....

....

....

....

....

BABY NOTES
(WHAT YOU DID, LOVED, NEEDED)

....

....

....

....

....

....

....

....

....

....

....

....

....

FEEDING NOTES
(TIME, DURATION/AMOUNT)

....

....

....

....

....

....

....

....

....

....

....

....

....

WELCOME TO
THE FOURTH TRIMESTER

WHAT IS IT?

The fourth trimester is the first 12 weeks of your baby's life and your new life as a mum. It's a time when you mimic your baby's environment inside the womb, outside. When you are encouraged to nurture your baby, as your body did before, with feeding, cuddling and soothing – without the fear that plagues so many new mums, of instilling bad habits. 'You can't spoil a newborn.' It's a crucial period for you both, where you treat those first three months in the way you treated your pregnancy. Preciously.

WHEN SOCIETY EXPECTS TOO MUCH

Beyond those first couple of weeks, there aren't many provisions for a new mum. All being well, your midwife signs you off at 10 days. Paternity leave ends. And you're left to your own devices. New mums are surrounded by so many pressures. The pressure to feel good. To look good. To have a baby who sleeps well. Feeds well. Settles well. And the frantic pace of life means that we almost expect these things to happen overnight. Add to this pressure hormonal changes and sleep deprivation and it's no wonder that so many new mums struggle in these first few months. But if you tapped into this fourth trimester lark, it could all be so different. You could relax a bit, cut yourself some slack and focus on the most important things of all: recovering and enjoying your baby.

YOU'VE JUST HAD A BABY

It might seem obvious: that after nine months of pregnancy it's going to take time to heal; that your baby is going to take time to adjust to the outside world. But for every rational thought like that, there's an irrational thought to counteract it. From sheer lack of sleep. From another mum whose baby is sleeping through at two weeks. From a book you read. From a well-meaning, passing comment that you look great when actually you feel dreadful. Anything that undermines you. That lulls you into a false reality when the reality is this: you've just had a baby.

SLOW DOWN

Remembering that there is a fourth trimester reminds you that in the first three months anything goes. You might feel good one day and rubbish the next. It's an unpredictable time and all you can do is live in each moment. And it's perfectly ok if you don't enjoy every moment. So try not to worry. Slow down. And stop rushing the whole process. Because the process is there for a reason.

HORMONES AND SLEEP DEPRIVATION

The physical trauma of pregnancy and birth is huge. We conveniently forget this because it's a 'natural' occurrence. Oestrogen levels play a big part in the way women feel after giving birth. After reaching a peak in the third trimester, in the 24 hours after labour they drop drastically and return to pre-pregnancy levels. If you're breastfeeding, your oestrogen levels remain low and you may experience symptoms such as night sweats, hot flashes, joint pain, mood swings, anxiety, depression, fatigue and insomnia. It helps to remember this. That there is an actual reason why you're waking up stuck to your duvet with a 1980s perm. Why you're feeling like you're losing the plot. You're not. And you won't be like this forever. You'll also be feeling sleep deprived. And there's little worse than sleep deprivation.

FEEL IT

Accept that you will feel up and down. Lower your expectations. Allow yourself to feel how you feel in any given moment. There's no need to pretend otherwise or put on a brave face. The fourth trimester is your friend. It's there to protect you. You can keep reminding yourself, 'I've just had a baby. Of course I'm going to feel like this.'

THIS TOO SHALL PASS

Nothing lasts forever. One day soon the tiny little baby you're holding in your arms will be a feisty toddler. Whilst this thought won't make you love them any more at 3.00AM, it might just make you cherish the fourth trimester for what it is. A permissible period of time to make the transition to motherhood. Not to mention 12 weeks of newborn cuddles, eating chocolate cake, wearing big pants and cutting yourself some serious slack. (Big pants optional.)

ON THIS DAY

DATE: _____

Give yourself a treat everyday. A nice coffee. A magazine. Or a slice of cake.

MY NOTES
(WHAT I LOVED, FELT, WISHED, NEEDED, STRUGGLED WITH, OVERCAME)

....

....

....

....

....

....

....

....

TO DO LIST

❑ ....

❑ ....

❑ ....

❑ ....

❑ ....

THINGS TO REMEMBER
(BECAUSE A BABY ATE MY BRAIN)

....
....
....
....
....

MEMORIES TO RECALL
(YEARS FROM NOW)

....
....
....
....
....

BABY NOTES
(WHAT YOU DID, LOVED, NEEDED)

....
....
....
....
....
....
....
....
....
....
....
....
....

FEEDING NOTES
(TIME, DURATION/AMOUNT)

....
....
....
....
....
....
....
....
....
....
....
....
....

STOP WORRYING.
SLOW DOWN.
REMEMBER.
YOU'VE JUST HAD
A BABY.

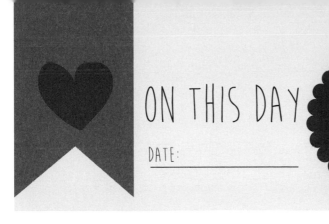

ON THIS DAY

DATE: _____

MY NOTES
(WHAT I LOVED, FELT, WISHED, NEEDED, STRUGGLED WITH, OVERCAME)

....

....

....

....

....

....

....

....

....

....

....

....

TO DO LIST

❏ ....

❏ ....

❏ ....

❏ ....

❏ ....

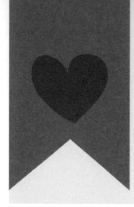

ON THIS DAY

DATE: _____

Take any offers of help. Food. Tidying up. Running errands. There are no prizes for flying solo.

MY NOTES
(WHAT I LOVED, FELT, WISHED, NEEDED, STRUGGLED WITH, OVERCAME)

....

....

....

....

....

....

....

....

....

....

....

TO DO LIST

☐ ....

☐ ....

☐ ....

☐ ....

☐ ....

THINGS TO REMEMBER
(BECAUSE A BABY ATE MY BRAIN)

....

....

....

....

....

MEMORIES TO RECALL
(YEARS FROM NOW)

....

....

....

....

....

BABY NOTES
(WHAT YOU DID, LOVED, NEEDED)

....

....

....

....

....

....

....

....

....

....

....

....

....

FEEDING NOTES
(TIME, DURATION/AMOUNT)

....

....

....

....

....

....

....

....

....

....

....

....

....

WOW!

YOU'VE SURVIVED THE FIRST MONTH. HOW AMAZING ARE YOU?

WHAT I'M MOST PROUD OF SO FAR:

....

....

....

....

....

....

MONTH TWO

Let's talk
about
SLEEP.

YOU WILL SLEEP AGAIN

THE SLEEP BANK

Sleep. It's pretty much the only thing you really know about having a baby – that you probably won't be getting much. During the second month with your baby you will notice that the sleep deprivation accumulates. This is likely to make you feel foggy, forgetful and probably a bit grumpy and teary. Make sure you implement some things to help you through. A nap during the day. IF YOU CAN. Go to bed after your baby's bedtime feed, before the next one is due. Or have someone else give this to them.

CONSERVE. CONSERVE. CONSERVE

The fourth trimester really comes into its own at this point. Because if you've been up half the night, why on earth would you want to do anything else but rest the next day? Resting (even if you're not actually sleeping) is crucial in helping to conserve your energy for the night ahead. So do lots of it. And watch all those box sets you've been meaning to catch up on.

IT'S OK TO HATE THE NIGHTFEED

It's 3.00AM. You're asleep. The type of sleep that borders on being knocked out, you're that tired. Suddenly you're awake. Just like that. There's a snuffle next to you. It starts off innocently enough. So you shut your eyes tight. If you go back to sleep, this will go away. But instead it builds up to a single cough. Your muscles contort in anticipation. 'Please, just let me sleep,' you think. It reaches a hacking cough. All you want is sleep. Then a wail. It's over, as it crescendos into a full-blown cry. No one really enjoys the night feeds. And that's ok. You aren't a badger, after all. It's also fine if the night feed makes you want to cry, utter profanities, slam doors and plot leaving your other half.

YOU WILL SLEEP AGAIN

I know it doesn't feel like it right now, but you WILL sleep again. As your baby grows and needs fewer feeds, the stretches of sleep will get longer. Remember this and don't get hung up on what another mum's baby is doing. Every baby is different. They do things in their own time. And also – sometimes – other mums exaggerate. Which doesn't make anyone feel better.

FILMS AND BOX SETS TO FEED BY

One of the perks of having a new baby is all the TV you get to watch. Guilt free. Here's a selection of films and box sets to feed by.

MUM RATING

TEAR JERKER
Feel-good film
but likely
to make you cry
(hormone
dependent)

MOOD LIFTER
Guaranteed to
make you
laugh/smile

ESCAPISM
For when you want
to escape
everyday life

WARNING
Graphic or complex
storylines
(not recommended
for the very
sleep-deprived)

FILMS

- About Time
- Begin Again
- Boyhood
- Bridesmaids
- Eat, Pray, Love
- Marley and Me
- Mona Lisa Smile
- Life as we know it
- Pride
- Sex and the City
- Steel Magnolias
- The Best Exotic Marigold Hotel
- The Best of Me
- The Fault in Our Stars
- The Odd Life of Timothy Green
- This is 40
- Up in the Air
- Walking on Sunshine
- We Bought a Zoo
- Where the Heart Is
- 500 Days Of Summer

BOX SETS

- Bomb Girls
- Breaking Bad
- Catastrophe
- Damages
- Desperate Housewives
- Game of Thrones
- Gossip Girl
- Grey's Anatomy
- Luther
- Mad Men
- Made in Chelsea
- New Girl
- Orange is the New Black
- Pramface
- Scandal
- Sex and the City
- The Affair
- The Big Bang Theory
- The Gilmore Girls
- The Real Housewives of Orange County/New York

BABY CINEMA

You can also catch all the new releases WITH your baby in tow.
Picturehouse cinemas host Big Scream and Odeon cinemas host Newbies –
your local cinema is sure to do similar parent and baby screenings.
Visit their websites for more information.

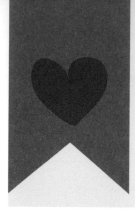

ON THIS DAY

DATE: _____

If it feels like you're always feeding, put on a box set. And make the most of sitting down.

MY NOTES
(WHAT I LOVED, FELT, WISHED, NEEDED, STRUGGLED WITH, OVERCAME)

....

....

....

....

....

....

....

....

....

....

....

....

TO DO LIST

❏ ....

❏ ....

❏ ....

❏ ....

❏ ....

THINGS TO REMEMBER
(BECAUSE A BABY ATE MY BRAIN)

....

....

....

....

....

MEMORIES TO RECALL
(YEARS FROM NOW)

....

....

....

....

....

BABY NOTES
(WHAT YOU DID, LOVED, NEEDED)

....

....

....

....

....

....

....

....

....

....

....

....

....

FEEDING NOTES
(TIME, DURATION/AMOUNT)

....

....

....

....

....

....

....

....

....

....

....

....

....

YOUR BABY.
YOUR RULES.

(never let anyone tell you
otherwise. Because no one
else knows your baby
like you do.)

ON THIS DAY

DATE: _____

Not every mum bonds with their baby instantly. Trust that it will come. Because it will.

MY NOTES
(WHAT I lOVED, FELT, WISHED, NEEDED, STRUGGLED WITH, OVERCAME)

....

....

....

....

....

....

....

....

....

....

....

TO DO LIST

❏ ....

❏ ....

❏ ....

❏ ....

❏ ....

ON THIS DAY

DATE: _____

You will doubt yourself A LOT. That's normal. Know that you're doing GREAT.

MY NOTES
(WHAT I LOVED, FELT, WISHED, NEEDED, STRUGGLED WITH, OVERCAME)

....

....

....

....

....

....

....

TO DO LIST

☐ ....

☐ ....

....

☐ ....

....

☐ ....

....

☐ ....

....

THINGS TO REMEMBER
(BECAUSE A BABY ATE MY BRAIN)

....
....
....
....
....

MEMORIES TO RECALL
(YEARS FROM NOW)

....
....
....
....
....

BABY NOTES
(WHAT YOU DID, LOVED, NEEDED)

....
....
....
....
....
....
....
....
....
....
....
....
....

FEEDING NOTES
(TIME, DURATION/AMOUNT)

....
....
....
....
....
....
....
....
....
....
....
....
....

☐ NEWBORN
☐ BIG PANTS
☐ SLAB OF CAKE
☐ BOXSET

(and that's today sorted.)

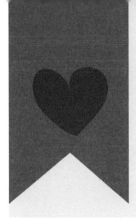

ON THIS DAY

DATE: _____

Dress your baby in comfy babygros. There's plenty of time to wear outfits.

MY NOTES
(WHAT I LOVED, FELT, WISHED, NEEDED, STRUGGLED WITH, OVERCAME)

....

....

....

....

....

....

....

....

....

....

....

....

TO DO LIST

❑ ....

❑ ....

❑ ....

❑ ....

❑ ....

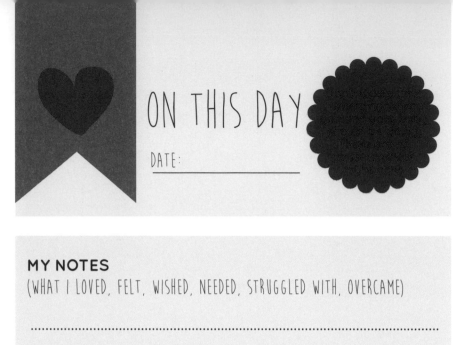

ON THIS DAY

DATE: _____

MY NOTES
(WHAT I LOVED, FELT, WISHED, NEEDED, STRUGGLED WITH, OVERCAME)

....

....

....

....

....

....

....

....

....

....

....

TO DO LIST

☐ ....

☐ ....

☐ ....

☐ ....

☐ ....

THINGS TO REMEMBER
(BECAUSE A BABY ATE MY BRAIN)

....
....
....
....
....

MEMORIES TO RECALL
(YEARS FROM NOW)

....
....
....
....
....

BABY NOTES
(WHAT YOU DID, LOVED, NEEDED)

....
....
....
....
....
....
....
....
....
....
....
....
....

FEEDING NOTES
(TIME, DURATION/AMOUNT)

....
....
....
....
....
....
....
....
....
....
....
....
....

TO ROUTINE OR NOT TO ROUTINE?

When I had my first baby I spent a lot of time wondering what sort of mother I wanted to be. An on demand, earth mother type? Or a routine type? I read a few contradictory books and attempted earth mothering whilst knowing deep down my personality was much better suited to being a routine mum. Cue lots of worrying, guilt and general confusion.

Three babies later, I now know that the first three months are NOT the time to be making these decisions. Having a rough feeding pattern is helpful (if only so you know you've fed your baby) but, beyond that, just be led by your baby's needs and your own. I've heard of mums waking their perfectly content, full babies because a certain routine says they must. 'Never wake a sleeping baby.'

There's plenty of time to decide what type of mother you would like to be. What sort of routine, if any, best suits your family. But it's not now. So put down the baby manuals and rest assured that whatever you are doing now is NOT setting a precedent for the future. It takes ONLY three days to change a habit.

Those first three months, that special fourth trimester, is like a honeymoon (without the beach and Pina Coloda). So make the most of it. Cuddle your baby as much as you like. Let them sleep on your chest. Savour them. Because the biggest cliché of all – that time passes so quickly – is not a cliché at all.

It's the truth.

NEW MUM'S SUPERFOOD SALAD

It's so difficult to find time to eat when you're a new mum. Chances are, when you do get a moment, you'll reach for something convenient, like a cake or biscuit. Now, I'm a BIG fan of cake and biscuits and totally encourage you to enjoy these. But if you're craving something nutritious, keep some of this easy, vitamin-charged salad in the fridge. If you roast a large sweet potato, this will last you 3-4 meals. You can keep all the ingredients in the fridge and then assemble in just five minutes when you want to eat. Better still, get someone else to do it for you! I've made all manner of versions of this salad, so improvise with squash, carrot, cheddar or whatever you have available!

INGREDIENTS (MAKES 3-4 PORTIONS)

Bag of spinach leaves

One avocado, sliced

A dozen baby tomatoes, halved

1 sweet potato, cubed and roasted

Sprinkle of feta/goat's cheese

Olive oil/Caesar salad dressing

Handful of nuts/sunflower seeds
(whatever you have in the cupboard)

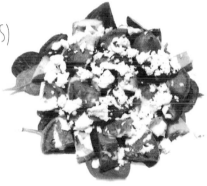

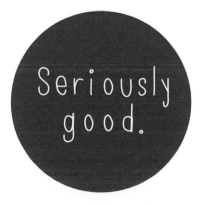

Seriously good.

METHOD

Roast the sweet potato in some olive oil at 180c for 25 minutes, until it's cooked. Assemble the spinach leaves on a plate. Add the tomatoes and avocado. Top with the roasted potato and the cheese. Drizzle with dressing and sprinkle with nuts or seeds. Serve with some wholemeal or seeded bread for a bit more bulk.

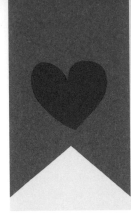

ON THIS DAY

DATE: _____

If your baby's feeding well, there's no need to wake them. They'll let you know when they're hungry!

MY NOTES
(WHAT I LOVED, FELT, WISHED, NEEDED, STRUGGLED WITH, OVERCAME)

....

....

....

....

....

....

....

....

....

....

TO DO LIST

☐ ....

☐ ....

☐ ....

☐ ....

☐ ....

THINGS TO REMEMBER
(BECAUSE A BABY ATE MY BRAIN)

....

....

....

....

....

MEMORIES TO RECALL
(YEARS FROM NOW)

....

....

....

....

....

BABY NOTES
(WHAT YOU DID, LOVED, NEEDED)

....

....

....

....

....

....

....

....

....

....

....

....

....

FEEDING NOTES
(TIME, DURATION/AMOUNT)

....

....

....

....

....

....

....

....

....

....

....

....

....

NEVER worry about
what you and your baby
SHOULD be doing.
You're already
doing EVERYTHING
you both need.

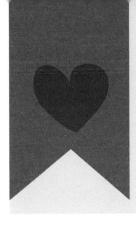

ON THIS DAY

DATE: _____

Meet a friend for coffee. Being with others is a natural mood lifter (even if getting out is an effort).

MY NOTES
(WHAT I LOVED, FELT, WISHED, NEEDED, STRUGGLED WITH, OVERCAME)

....

....

....

....

....

....

....

....

....

....

....

TO DO LIST

☐ ....

☐ ....

☐ ....

☐ ....

☐ ....

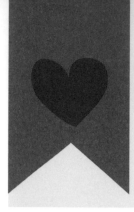

ON THIS DAY

DATE: _____

Feeling tired? Get your head down. A quick recharge can do wonders. Everything else will wait.

MY NOTES
(WHAT I LOVED, FELT, WISHED, NEEDED, STRUGGLED WITH, OVERCAME)

....

....

....

....

....

....

....

....

....

....

....

TO DO LIST

❑ ....

❑ ....

❑ ....

❑ ....

❑ ....

THINGS TO REMEMBER
(BECAUSE A BABY ATE MY BRAIN)

....
....
....
....
....

MEMORIES TO RECALL
(YEARS FROM NOW)

....
....
....
....
....

BABY NOTES
(WHAT YOU DID, LOVED, NEEDED)

....
....
....
....
....
....
....
....
....
....
....
....
....

FEEDING NOTES
(TIME, DURATION/AMOUNT)

....
....
....
....
....
....
....
....
....
....
....
....
....

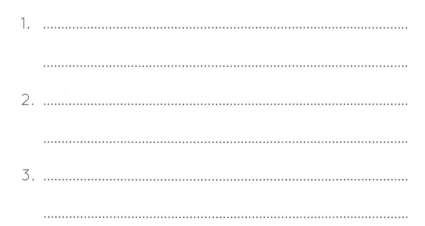

TWO MONTHS OLD ALREADY! YOU'RE TOTALLY ROCKING THIS MOTHERHOOD LARK.

THREE THINGS I'VE ACHIEVED THIS MONTH:

1. ....
....

2. ....
....

3. ....
....

MONTH THREE

Don't
be afraid
to ask for
help.

YOU'RE STILL A NEW MUM

AN IMPORTANT REMINDER

Around the third month, others can forget that you're still very much a new mum. You, yourself, may forget this because your newborn isn't so new anymore. They might be smiling. And in the next size babygro already. To that hectic outside world, you're doing ok. Your baby is bouncing, you've brushed your hair and you're dressed (sort of). Yet some days, nothing could be further from the truth. Because looking after a baby is such a fine balance between coping and chaos. It depends on so many factors. Mostly SLEEP. So you need to continue to take time to rest and not take on board other people's expectations.

OFFERING HELP AND ASKING FOR HELP

If the offers of help have dwindled, don't be afraid to ask for what you need. No one expects you to do this huge task of looking after a tiny human being on your own. Remember, they've just got caught up in their own, busy lives. Ask a friend to have the baby for an hour. Let your other half know you need them to take over the chores or cooking. Don't be afraid to ask. You're not failing if you do.

HAVING A NEW BABY IS LONELY

With new babies come demands. Demands that take you away from the outside world, that is having a far better life than you currently are. Or ever will again. Parties. Nights out. Holidays. All documented by the wonder that is social media. When you're tired and struggling – all normal terrain with a new baby in tow – these things can become magnified and make you feel like you're on your own. It's a sign you need looking after. A check-in from a friend. A hug from your other half. A hot dinner. Any gesture that says, 'You're not alone. You're loved.' (Also, they're not really having a better life than you. It just feels like that right now).

DON'T DOUBT YOURSELF

If it's your first baby, you'll spend a lot of time doubting yourself. A LOT. You'll worry that your baby isn't a) feeding enough b) sleeping enough c) doing somersaults yet. Are they developing normally? Why is your friend's baby doing X when yours can't even do Y? WHY?, WHY?, WHY? If it's your second, third, or fourth baby, you'll still spend a lot of time doubting yourself. Except this time you'll feel like a fraud. Because it's your second, third or fourth baby. You know what you're doing. This should be easy by now. But every baby is different. In that respect, every baby may as well be the first. When it comes to having a baby, we're all new mums. No matter what round we're on.

FEELINGS OF FAILURE

Guilt and feelings of failure unfortunately come with the territory of being a mum (more in Month Nine). It's especially normal to experience these feelings very profoundly with an unexpected, traumatic birth or trouble breastfeeding. Allow yourself to feel sad and disappointed that labour didn't go how you thought it would go. Then get some help in processing this from a health professional, so you can understand what happened and why. And start to resolve it in your own mind. Similarly with breastfeeding, if it wasn't for you for whatever reason, make peace with that now. And remember, there's more than one way to skin a cat. Never, ever believe you've failed because things turned out differently than you imagined. How could you have done? You've made and are nurturing that lovely, little baby staring back at you.

ONE DAY AT A TIME

In the darkness of a 3.00 AM night feed, it can all feel relentless. Right now it is pretty relentless. But it WILL get easier. One day at a time. So live in the moment and don't fast forward to further down the line. This can be a scary, unknown place that only adds to the overwhelming sense of responsibility you already feel. Get there when you get there. Instead, breathe. And breathe some more. Then remember, this is the most challenging thing you'll ever do. You don't need to be doing better. You're already good enough.

A NOTE

It's perfectly normal to feel lonely, low or up and down when you've had a baby. We've all been there, I promise you. Getting that elusive 'rest' can help, so can a good(ish) diet and gentle exercise (a walk with a pram, not a marathon). But if you're ever concerned that your feelings are becoming a little too low, please speak to someone who knows you well or your GP. There's more on post-natal depression in Month Four.

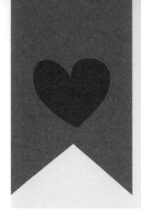

ON THIS DAY

DATE: _____

You've possibly had your post-natal check. But there's still a way to go. Take things slow.

MY NOTES
(WHAT I LOVED, FELT, WISHED, NEEDED, STRUGGLED WITH, OVERCAME)

....

....

....

....

....

....

....

TO DO LIST

❑ ....

❑ ....

❑ ....

❑ ....

❑ ....

THINGS TO REMEMBER
(BECAUSE A BABY ATE MY BRAIN)

....

....

....

....

....

MEMORIES TO RECALL
(YEARS FROM NOW)

....

....

....

....

....

BABY NOTES
(WHAT YOU DID, LOVED, NEEDED)

....

....

....

....

....

....

....

....

....

....

....

....

....

FEEDING NOTES
(TIME, DURATION/AMOUNT)

....

....

....

....

....

....

....

....

....

....

....

....

....

HAPPY MUM
=
HAPPY BABY
SO DON'T BEAT
YOURSELF UP
ABOUT ANYTHING.

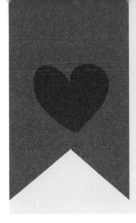

ON THIS DAY

DATE: _____

Don't compare yourself to other mums. Who could be better for your baby than you?

MY NOTES
(WHAT I LOVED, FELT, WISHED, NEEDED, STRUGGLED WITH, OVERCAME)

....

....

....

....

....

....

....

....

....

....

....

TO DO LIST

❏ ....

❏ ....

❏ ....

❏ ....

❏ ....

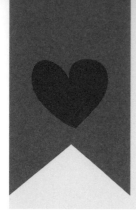

ON THIS DAY

DATE: _____

If exercising, take it easy. A gentle walk. Or join a buggy fit class and meet other mums.

MY NOTES
(WHAT I LOVED, FELT, WISHED, NEEDED, STRUGGLED WITH, OVERCAME)

....

....

....

....

....

....

....

....

....

....

....

TO DO LIST

❑ ....

❑ ....

❑ ....

❑ ....

❑ ....

THINGS TO REMEMBER
(BECAUSE A BABY ATE MY BRAIN)

....

....

....

....

....

MEMORIES TO RECALL
(YEARS FROM NOW)

....

....

....

....

....

BABY NOTES
(WHAT YOU DID, LOVED, NEEDED)

....

....

....

....

....

....

....

....

....

....

....

....

....

FEEDING NOTES
(TIME, DURATION/AMOUNT)

....

....

....

....

....

....

....

....

....

....

....

....

....

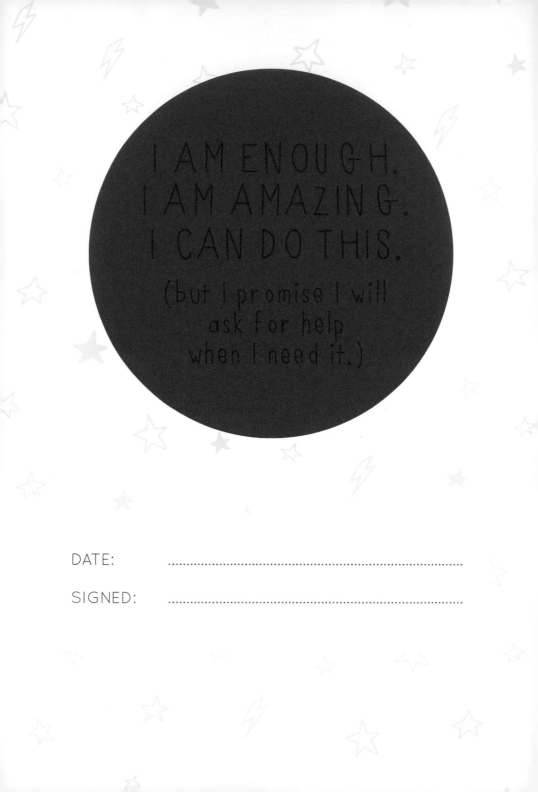

I AM ENOUGH.
I AM AMAZING.
I CAN DO THIS.
(but I promise I will
ask for help
when I need it..)

DATE: ....

SIGNED: ....

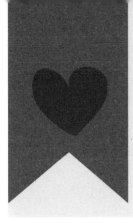

ON THIS DAY

DATE: _____

Worried your baby isn't getting enough stimulation? Don't. You and your world are plenty.

MY NOTES
(WHAT I LOVED, FELT, WISHED, NEEDED, STRUGGLED WITH, OVERCAME)

....

....

....

....

....

....

....

....

....

....

....

....

TO DO LIST

❑ ....

❑ ....

❑ ....

❑ ....

❑ ....

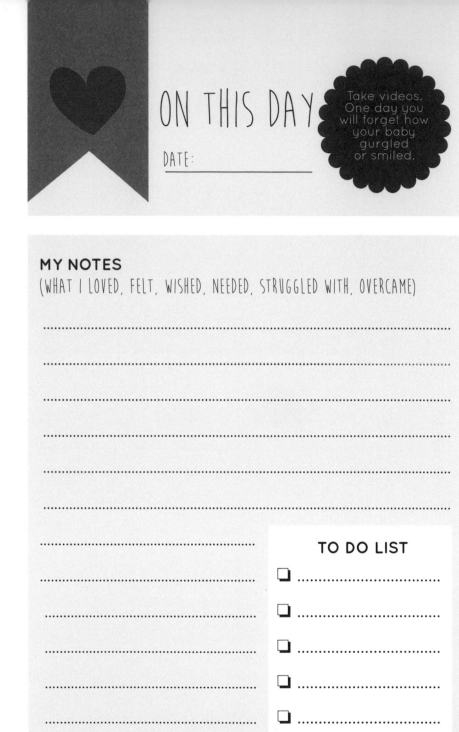

ON THIS DAY

DATE: _____

Take videos.
One day you
will forget how
your baby
gurgled
or smiled.

MY NOTES
(WHAT I LOVED, FELT, WISHED, NEEDED, STRUGGLED WITH, OVERCAME)

....

....

....

....

....

....

....

....

....

....

TO DO LIST

☐ ....

☐ ....

☐ ....

☐ ....

☐ ....

THINGS TO REMEMBER
(BECAUSE A BABY ATE MY BRAIN)

....
....
....
....
....

MEMORIES TO RECALL
(YEARS FROM NOW)

....
....
....
....
....

BABY NOTES
(WHAT YOU DID, LOVED, NEEDED)

....
....
....
....
....
....
....
....
....
....
....
....
....

FEEDING NOTES
(TIME, DURATION/AMOUNT)

....
....
....
....
....
....
....
....
....
....
....
....
....

'NO SEX PLEASE. WE'RE PARENTS'

You've had your post-natal check and, if your labour was straight-forward and everything is healing as it should, your nurse probably asked you about contraception and whether you're having sex. 'Sex?' you cry. 'Are you kidding me?'

Your other half, on the other hand, has possibly already brought the subject up. Once or twice. In a tentative, 'Don't anger her, just kidding,' sort of way when they see the horrified reaction on your face.

Having sex after a baby is, let's be frank here, scary. A bit weird. No one relishes the thought. You're bruised and battered and, even if you're not, emotionally you're just not there yet. Sleep deprivation and the non-randy kind of hormones don't exactly make for a romantic encounter. Sooner or later you'll want/need to get back on the horse, so to speak, but it's important you feel comfortable about when this happens. Like everything else, there's no rush.

Whenever you do decide the time is right, this is another occasion NOT to compare yourself to others. Some mums wait a few weeks. Others go an entire year. Whatever the case is for you, the first time after a baby will be a bit functional. And you'll probably breathe a sigh of relief when it's over. That's perfectly normal. No one expects you to be swinging from the chandeliers. (Good on you if you do though.)

And if you have a bunch of awesome new mum friends, don't be afraid to bring this subject up. Once someone's brave enough to ask the question, you'll all be chipping in.

And having a good laugh whilst you do.

NEW MUM'S CHOCOLATE FRIDGE CAKE

Why have sex when you can have chocolate? Why, indeed. This recipe is super-easy and so delicious that you'll only make the mistake of sharing it once. The cocoa content in dark chocolate is a natural mood enhancer and also contains magnesium, which improves neurological and muscle function that can be easily depleted in women. In other words? This fridge cake is GOOD for you. Also, you can make this with whatever you have in the cupboard. Apricots, nuts, cereal – it all works!

INGREDIENTS

250g/8oz digestive biscuits
150g/5oz milk chocolate
150g/5oz dark chocolate
100g/3oz unsalted butter
150g/5oz golden syrup
2 handfuls of mini marshmallows
75g/2oz raisins

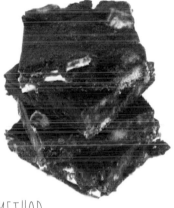

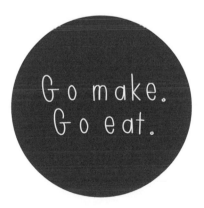

Go make.
Go eat.

METHOD

Line a shallow tin with cling film. Bash the digestives in a sandwich bag with a rolling pin. Melt the chocolate, butter and golden syrup in a bowl over a pan of simmering water, stirring occasionally. Remove from heat and stir in the biscuit pieces, raisins and marshmallows. Spoon mixture into tin and level. Cool in the fridge for 2 hours. Turn the mixture out, peel off cling film and cut into squares (or eat the whole thing in one go).

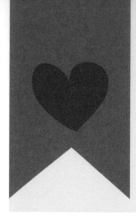

ON THIS DAY

DATE: _____

Every day is different. If today was hard, believe that tomorrow may be easier.

MY NOTES
(WHAT I LOVED, FELT, WISHED, NEEDED, STRUGGLED WITH, OVERCAME)

....

....

....

....

....

....

....

....

....

....

....

TO DO LIST

❏ ....

❏ ....

❏ ....

❏ ....

❏ ....

THINGS TO REMEMBER
(BECAUSE A BABY ATE MY BRAIN)

....

....

....

....

....

MEMORIES TO RECALL
(YEARS FROM NOW)

....

....

....

....

....

BABY NOTES
(WHAT YOU DID, LOVED, NEEDED)

....

....

....

....

....

....

....

....

....

....

....

....

....

....

FEEDING NOTES
(TIME, DURATION/AMOUNT)

....

....

....

....

....

....

....

....

....

....

....

....

....

....

Motherhood
can be hard.
Be that mum
who opens up.
(see what happens.)

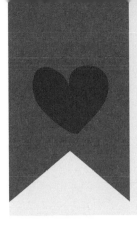

ON THIS DAY

DATE: _____

Take some time for you. Light a candle. Breathe deeply. Be calm. If only for a moment.

MY NOTES
(WHAT I LOVED, FELT, WISHED, NEEDED, STRUGGLED WITH, OVERCAME)

....

....

....

....

....

....

....

....

....

....

....

TO DO LIST

❏ ....

❏ ....

❏ ....

❏ ....

❏ ....

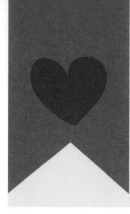

ON THIS DAY

DATE: _____

Feeling the pressure to be back to normal? Ask yourself this. 'What's the rush, really?'

MY NOTES
(WHAT I LOVED, FELT, WISHED, NEEDED, STRUGGLED WITH, OVERCAME)

....

....

....

....

....

....

....

....

....

....

....

TO DO LIST

☐ ....

☐ ....

☐ ....

☐ ....

☐ ....

THINGS TO REMEMBER
(BECAUSE A BABY ATE MY BRAIN)

....

....

....

....

....

MEMORIES TO RECALL
(YEARS FROM NOW)

....

....

....

....

....

BABY NOTES
(WHAT YOU DID, LOVED, NEEDED)

....

....

....

....

....

....

....

....

....

....

....

....

....

FEEDING NOTES
(TIME, DURATION/AMOUNT)

....

....

....

....

....

....

....

....

....

....

....

....

....

YOU'VE MADE THE FOURTH TRIMESTER!

And you're ready
for whatever comes next.
(as long as there's cake.)

MY THREE GOALS GOING FORWARD:

1. ....

....

2. ....

....

3. ....

....

MONTH FOUR

Look
after
yourself.

LET'S TALK ABOUT POST-NATAL DEPRESSION

IN YOUR OWN TIME

The fourth trimester may be over but this doesn't mean you should suddenly feel the pressure to be firing on all cylinders again. You still have a new baby and may continue to wear big pants and eat cake for as long as you like. And I hope you do.

HOW ARE YOU FEELING?

Around this time, some mums may be thriving. Others, not so much. Some might even be feeling beside themselves and that can often be an indication that things aren't quite right. So, let's talk a little bit about post-natal depression (PND). Because it shouldn't be something we're scared of or afraid to mention. It does happen, unfortunately, but it can be treated very effectively and the sooner it's diagnosed, the better. All new mums deserve to understand what to look out for because it can be difficult to know when you're a mum for the very first time. How are you supposed to feel?

WHAT IS PND?

PND is very different to the baby blues, which most, if not all, women experience in the first couple of weeks after birth as their hormones literally crash. It is also more than feeling tired or occasionally low. PND is different for everyone, but typical symptoms include frequent tearfulness, anxiety of any form (health anxiety is common), panic (may include panic attacks), insomnia, extreme lethargy, trouble bonding with your baby (or detaching yourself from any other children) and a sense of doom or hopelessness. It can also manifest itself very physically with muscle aches, headaches and a general state of feeling unwell, leading new mums to think it must be something serious (that's usually the health anxiety talking). Because what a lot of people don't know is that when you're very depressed, you can actually feel it physically. Another common factor is an overwhelming feeling that you just can't cope – often with things that never fathomed you before. It might be getting up in the morning. Dressing yourself and your baby. Doing the nursery/school run, if you have other children. You just can't seem to manage it.

'HOW DO I KNOW?'

One of the cruellest things about PND is that when you're in it you can't really see you're in it. You know you're in a fog. You know you feel the worst you've ever felt. 'But I've got a baby,' you reason, 'I'm not going to feel amazing, am I?' Well actually, yes, you have got a baby but, no, you shouldn't feel like that. At this point, the support of someone who knows you really well is helpful. Someone you can turn to and say, 'I'm really, really struggling. Do *you* think I'm struggling?'

YOU CAN DO THIS

I'm not ashamed PND happened to me after my third baby. It was nothing I did. With a combination of antidepressants and Cognitive Behavioural Therapy (CBT) counselling, I now have coping mechanisms I never would have developed without it. PND isn't a pleasant experience but the good news is you do get through it, once you get help. If you suspect you may have PND, speak to your doctor (ask them to do a full blood count to rule out any other cause). They can discuss treatment with you, which may take the form of counselling or a combination of counselling and medication. Don't be afraid of medication if this is recommended to you. You haven't failed. It isn't your fault. Sometimes after birth the hormones are a bit wonky and your body fails to produce enough of the happy hormone, serotonin, so you need a little help. Either way, things won't improve overnight but a few weeks in you'll start to feel a bit more like you. Be patient with yourself. Recovery does take time. But you WILL get better.

SOME USEFUL READING
APNI (Association of Post-Natal Illness)
www.apni.org
They have some comprehensive online leaflets, which I found very helpful, and you can also call them to be put in touch with someone who has recovered from PND. Hearing positive stories can be very reassuring.

You can read more about my personal story at Surviving Motherhood: 'Me and PND'.

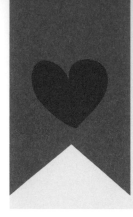

ON THIS DAY

DATE: _____

If you ever feel like you're sinking, tell someone you trust.

MY NOTES
(WHAT I LOVED, FELT, WISHED, NEEDED, STRUGGLED WITH, OVERCAME)

....

....

....

....

....

....

....

....

....

....

....

TO DO LIST

❑ ....

❑ ....

❑ ....

❑ ....

❑ ....

THINGS TO REMEMBER
(BECAUSE A BABY ATE MY BRAIN)

....
....
....
....
....

MEMORIES TO RECALL
(YEARS FROM NOW)

....
....
....
....
....

BABY NOTES
(WHAT YOU DID, LOVED, NEEDED)

....
....
....
....
....
....
....
....
....
....
....
....
....

FEEDING NOTES
(TIME, DURATION/AMOUNT)

....
....
....
....
....
....
....
....
....
....
....
....
....

We only worry about the past or the future. So try and be present in the moment that's happening NOW.

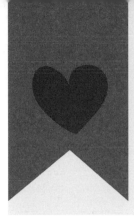

ON THIS DAY

DATE: _____

Got new mum friends? Set up a weekly meet. Someone will always turn up. With cake.

MY NOTES
(WHAT I lOVED, FELT, WISHED, NEEDED, STRUGGLED WITH, OVERCAME)

....

....

....

....

....

....

....

....

....

....

....

TO DO LIST

❑ ....

❑ ....

❑ ....

❑ ....

❑ ....

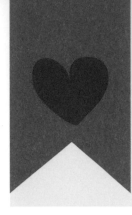

ON THIS DAY

DATE:

Had a bad night? Acknowledge you feel rubbish and lower your expectations.

MY NOTES
(WHAT I LOVED, FELT, WISHED, NEEDED, STRUGGLED WITH, OVERCAME)

....

....

....

....

....

....

....

....

....

....

....

TO DO LIST

❏ ....

❏ ....

❏ ....

❏ ....

❏ ....

THINGS TO REMEMBER
(BECAUSE A BABY ATE MY BRAIN)

....
....
....
....
....

MEMORIES TO RECALL
(YEARS FROM NOW)

....
....
....
....
....

BABY NOTES
(WHAT YOU DID, LOVED, NEEDED)

....
....
....
....
....
....
....
....
....
....
....
....
....

FEEDING NOTES
(TIME, DURATION/AMOUNT)

....
....
....
....
....
....
....
....
....
....
....
....
....

I HAVE A DUTY TO
LOOK AFTER MYSELF
AND I TAKE THIS
DUTY SERIOUSLY.

(remind yourself
when you forget.)

DATE: ....

SIGNED: ....

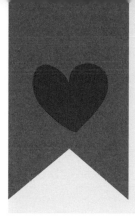

ON THIS DAY

DATE: _____

Don't feel bad if you find yourself wishing some days away. That's normal.

MY NOTES
(WHAT I LOVED, FELT, WISHED, NEEDED, STRUGGLED WITH, OVERCAME)

....

....

....

....

....

....

....

....

....

....

....

TO DO LIST

❑ ....

❑ ....

❑ ....

❑ ....

❑ ....

ON THIS DAY

DATE: _____

Go shopping. Treat yourself. It won't be as easy when your baby's moving.

MY NOTES
(WHAT I LOVED, FELT, WISHED, NEEDED, STRUGGLED WITH, OVERCAME)

....

....

....

....

....

....

....

TO DO LIST

- [ ] ....
- [ ] ....
- [ ] ....
- [ ] ....
- [ ] ....

THINGS TO REMEMBER
(BECAUSE A BABY ATE MY BRAIN)

....

....

....

....

....

MEMORIES TO RECALL
(YEARS FROM NOW)

....

....

....

....

....

BABY NOTES
(WHAT YOU DID, LOVED, NEEDED)

....

....

....

....

....

....

....

....

....

....

....

....

....

FEEDING NOTES
(TIME, DURATION/AMOUNT)

....

....

....

....

....

....

....

....

....

....

....

....

....

HAVE A HEALTHY MIND

There are some simple CBT techniques you can introduce to help yourself have a healthy, happy mind in those early months of motherhood. Here are a few that are well worth practicing on a daily basis, until they become second nature.

KNOW YOUR TRIGGERS

It is useful to know your personal triggers that can lead to you feeling low or sensitive. Because once you've acknowledged them, you can accept and rationalise how you're feeling. Common triggers include tiredness, hormones, habits such as worrying and spending too much time alone.

LIVE IN THE MOMENT

Initially, this is perhaps one of the most difficult things to do. We're so used to looking forward all the time, and often looking back. But once you're more able to stay in the present moment, you will find it eliminates most of the opportunity for worry. After all, we rarely worry about what's happening in the actual moment. We tend to focus our anxiety on what may happen in the future. So. If your baby's not sleeping, instead of focusing on the actual moment your mind fast forwards into the future and, before you know it, has suddenly reached the catastrophic conclusion that your baby will never sleep and you will be sleep deprived for the rest of time. DISASTER. If you stay in the moment, you only deal with what is happening now, which is the only part of life you can control anyway. This does take practice, but it's well worth persevering with because once you can do it, it's liberating.

MOMENTS PASS

'This too shall pass' is a very popular mantra in motherhood, meaning all moments pass – like that thing your baby's started doing that you wish they hadn't! Think of an occasion that challenged you. Did it last forever? Or, minutes later, were you experiencing something else? Life is a series of moments, some good, some challenging. Remember that nothing lasts forever and you will learn to tolerate the uncertainty of life. And motherhood.

CHALLENGE UNHELPFUL THOUGHTS

So often, what we believe to be true is based on fantasy. A fantasy that our minds have made up. A fantasy made up of lots of unhelpful thoughts. Thought challenging is basically thinking of a situation in a different, more helpful way. So to use the example of your baby not sleeping, instead of reaching the catastrophic thought that, 'Arggghhh, my baby is NEVER going to sleep! I can't go on like this!' you would instead challenge yourself to think about it differently. Perhaps like this. 'OK, my baby isn't sleeping today. But they're only small still. It won't be like this forever, but in the meantime we'll take it easy and watch a film.' So next time a catastrophic thought enters your mind ask yourself, 'Is this helpful? How can I think about this differently?'

FOCUS YOUR ATTENTION

This is a fabulous technique, especially for dealing with health anxiety. If I ask you to think about your left big toe, what happens? Are you suddenly really aware of it? Well, imagine the same with any part of your body. If your focus of attention is directed towards that headache, your stiff neck or the tightness in your chest, you will feel it even more. 'Living in the moment' and turning your attention to what's happening in the present can help with this. But it will take time retraining your mind. So be patient.

CBT YOUR WAY TO A HEALTHY MIND

1. KNOW YOUR TRIGGERS
2. LIVE IN THE MOMENT
3. CHALLENGE UNHELPFUL THOUGHTS
4. REFOCUS YOUR ATTENTION

For more information on CBT – what it can do for you and how to find a local practitioner – visit the MIND website: www.mind.org.uk

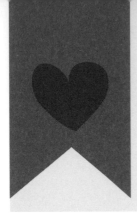

ON THIS DAY

DATE: _____

Always be patient with yourself. Motherhood is a steep learning curve.

MY NOTES
(WHAT I LOVED, FELT, WISHED, NEEDED, STRUGGLED WITH, OVERCAME)

....

....

....

....

....

....

....

....

....

....

....

TO DO LIST

❑ ....

❑ ....

❑ ....

❑ ....

❑ ....

THINGS TO REMEMBER
(BECAUSE A BABY ATE MY BRAIN)

....
....
....
....
....

MEMORIES TO RECALL
(YEARS FROM NOW)

....
....
....
....
....

BABY NOTES
(WHAT YOU DID, LOVED, NEEDED)

....
....
....
....
....
....
....
....
....
....
....
....
....

FEEDING NOTES
(TIME, DURATION/AMOUNT)

....
....
....
....
....
....
....
....
....
....
....
....
....

Every mum's
stood where you
stand now. And
every mum's
stepped beyond.

(it will get easier.)

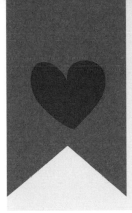

ON THIS DAY

DATE: _____

MY NOTES
(WHAT I LOVED, FELT, WISHED, NEEDED, STRUGGLED WITH, OVERCAME)

....

....

....

....

....

....

....

....

....

....

....

TO DO LIST

❑ ....

❑ ....

❑ ....

❑ ....

❑ ....

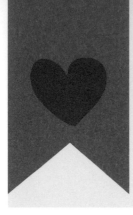

ON THIS DAY

DATE: _____

Try a Mum & Baby yoga class. Time to bond. And time for you.

MY NOTES
(WHAT I LOVED, FELT, WISHED, NEEDED, STRUGGLED WITH, OVERCAME)

....

....

....

....

....

....

....

....

....

....

....

TO DO LIST

❑ ....

❑ ....

❑ ....

❑ ....

❑ ....

THINGS TO REMEMBER
(BECAUSE A BABY ATE MY BRAIN)

....
....
....
....
....

MEMORIES TO RECALL
(YEARS FROM NOW)

....
....
....
....
....

BABY NOTES
(WHAT YOU DID, LOVED, NEEDED)

....
....
....
....
....
....
....
....
....
....
....
....
....

FEEDING NOTES
(TIME, DURATION/AMOUNT)

....
....
....
....
....
....
....
....
....
....
....
....
....

FOUR MONTHS!

ONE DAY YOU'LL LOOK BACK AND WISH YOU'D STOPPED TO TAKE A BREATH.

A MOMENT WHEN I TOOK THAT BREATH:

....

....

....

....

....

MONTH FIVE

Keep going.
You've got
this.

A LETTER TO A SLEEP-DEPRIVED MUM

Dear New Mum,

You may have been getting some sleep now that the newborn days are behind you, if your baby is sleeping longer stretches. But around the end of month four/the beginning of month five, many babies take advantage of the dreaded four month sleep regression, throwing you into a frenzy of worry and self-doubt. 'What am I doing wrong?' you'll think. NOTHING. This is simply a prelude to what comes next – your baby 'growing up' and going through some neurological changes. Many mums also find that it's a sign their baby is getting hungrier before weaning commences, usually around six months. So don't stress if your baby wants more milk in the lead-up to this. Just go with it and rest assured that things will have settled down by the time you introduce solids. You'll sleep again.

In the meantime, do NOT underestimate the effect of lack of sleep. Do NOT be hard on yourself. Do NOT ask yourself why you aren't coping better. Why you are crying at the silliest of things. Why you aren't the resilient woman you once were. YOU STILL ARE. In fact, you are more resilient than ever, because you now do far more on much less.

Sleep deprivation is cruel. It has you questioning everything. Forgetting your name. Who you are. BUT YOU ARE STILL YOU. And you will get through today. With lots of coffee. Some comforting words from a friend who gets it. And the hope that tonight you will sleep and tomorrow will be better.

Keep going. You're doing fine. I'm with you all the way.

Amy x

10 THINGS YOU CAN DO WHEN YOUR BABY REFUSES TO SLEEP

1. **Cry.** It's ok to mourn the sleep you so desperately miss.

2. **Calculate your baby's value on eBay.** Do NOT mention sleeping ability.

3. **Curse** all the neighbours whose houses are still in complete darkness.

4. **Prod your partner.** Stick things in their ears. Up their nose.

5. If that doesn't rouse them, **slam doors.**

6. **Check Facebook and Twitter repeatedly.** And connect with other insomniac mums.

7. **Spend money, online, for things you don't need.** (And things you'll forgot you even ordered, until they turn up).

8. **Eat breakfast at 5.00AM.** At least you're getting ahead of the day, right?

9. **Remember and laugh** at all the things you thought you'd 'achieve' on maternity leave. With all that time you were suddenly going to have.

10. **Nod off.** And repeat. For the rest of the day.

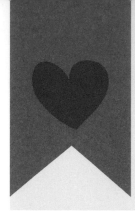

ON THIS DAY

DATE: _____

If sleep is off the agenda, remember the fourth trimester rules.

MY NOTES
(WHAT I LOVED, FELT, WISHED, NEEDED, STRUGGLED WITH, OVERCAME)

....

....

....

....

....

....

....

....

....

....

....

TO DO LIST

❑ ....

❑ ....

❑ ....

❑ ....

❑ ....

THINGS TO REMEMBER
(BECAUSE A BABY ATE MY BRAIN)

....
....
....
....
....

MEMORIES TO RECALL
(YEARS FROM NOW)

....
....
....
....
....

BABY NOTES
(WHAT YOU DID, LOVED, NEEDED)

....
....
....
....
....
....
....
....
....
....
....
....
....
....

FEEDING NOTES
(TIME, DURATION/AMOUNT)

....
....
....
....
....
....
....
....
....
....
....
....
....
....

The early bird might catch the worm. But the late bird gets a lie in and a bacon butty.

(try and nab a well-deserved lie-in one morning.)

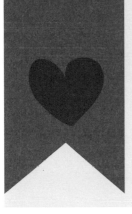

ON THIS DAY

DATE: _____

When you're tired, you need a break. Remember to ask for one.

MY NOTES
(WHAT I LOVED, FELT, WISHED, NEEDED, STRUGGLED WITH, OVERCAME)

....

....

....

....

....

....

....

....

....

....

....

TO DO LIST

❑ ....

❑ ....

❑ ....

❑ ....

❑ ....

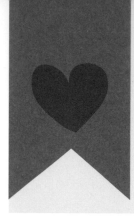

ON THIS DAY

DATE: _____

Nothing beats
Baby Cinema with
a bacon butty
and coffee.

MY NOTES
(WHAT I LOVED, FELT, WISHED, NEEDED, STRUGGLED WITH, OVERCAME)

....

....

....

....

....

....

....

....

....

....

....

TO DO LIST

❏ ....

❏ ....

❏ ....

❏ ....

❏ ....

THINGS TO REMEMBER
(BECAUSE A BABY ATE MY BRAIN)

....
....
....
....
....

MEMORIES TO RECALL
(YEARS FROM NOW)

....
....
....
....
....

BABY NOTES
(WHAT YOU DID, LOVED, NEEDED)

....
....
....
....
....
....
....
....
....
....
....
....
....
....

FEEDING NOTES
(TIME, DURATION/AMOUNT)

....
....
....
....
....
....
....
....
....
....
....
....
....
....

It is good for
me and my baby
to have time apart.
I will not feel guilty
for needing this.

DATE: ....

SIGNED: ....

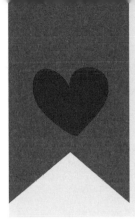

ON THIS DAY

DATE: _____

Always accept the moment as it is.

MY NOTES
(WHAT I LOVED, FELT, WISHED, NEEDED, STRUGGLED WITH, OVERCAME)

....

....

....

....

....

....

....

TO DO LIST

....

☐ ....

....

☐ ....

....

☐ ....

....

☐ ....

....

☐ ....

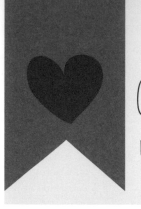

ON THIS DAY

Praise yourself for something you've done well today.

DATE: _____

MY NOTES
(WHAT I LOVED, FELT, WISHED, NEEDED, STRUGGLED WITH, OVERCAME)

....

....

....

....

....

....

....

....

....

....

....

TO DO LIST

❑ ....

❑ ....

❑ ....

❑ ....

❑ ....

THINGS TO REMEMBER
(BECAUSE A BABY ATE MY BRAIN)

....
....
....
....
....

MEMORIES TO RECALL
(YEARS FROM NOW)

....
....
....
....
....

BABY NOTES
(WHAT YOU DID, LOVED, NEEDED)

....
....
....
....
....
....
....
....
....
....
....
....
....

FEEDING NOTES
(TIME, DURATION/AMOUNT)

....
....
....
....
....
....
....
....
....
....
....
....
....

IT WILL GET EASIER

'REALLY? WHEN?'

You've probably noticed that others are often reassuring you and telling you, 'It will get easier'. Hopefully, things already are a little easier than those newborn days. But if they aren't, or the four month sleep regression is in full swing, these words will feel like a very empty gesture and may even leave you confused or filled with even more self-doubt. 'What am I doing wrong? Why isn't it easier?' are just some of the questions you might start asking yourself.

SLEEPING MORE

Not to state the obvious but as mums get more sleep, they often find it also gets easier. Simply because they have more resources and general well-being to tackle the day ahead. So. If you're not yet getting this precious sleep, cut yourself some serious slack and don't ask yourself when it will get easier. Just trust that, eventually, it will. And you never know. That 'eventually' may well be tomorrow. So keep going. You're doing great.

FEEDING LESS

Lots of mums find it becomes less relentless when their baby doesn't need quite so many feeds and they can consider having a break. During those early days, it feels like that's all you do. When you have fewer bottles or breastfeeds to worry about, this can give you a bigger window to leave your baby during the day.

TAKING A BREAK FROM YOUR BABY

Leaving your baby for the first time is always strange but it really is good for you both and can give you some much needed space to step out of the role of nurturer and nurture yourself for a change. You'll return feeling recharged with more energy and patience for you and your baby. Never feel guilty for taking this time, if and when you can. Likewise, never feel forced into leaving your baby by a well-meaning friend or relative, if you're not ready to do so, or simply don't feel the need for your own time right now. The key here is always doing whatever YOU are ready to do and not feeling guilty either way.

ACCEPTING EVERY STAGE

Just as some things get easier, some things get harder. This is the nature of being a mother – every stage is different. Your baby may start to sleep. But then they start crawling, which brings its own challenges for a period of time. It helps to remember this when you're navigating any stage of motherhood. Not only does it stop you wishing that stage away, but it can help restore a sense of calm and balance and remove that tendency to think catastrophic thoughts, leaving you to appreciate the moment. And trust that all will be, as it should be. In the end.

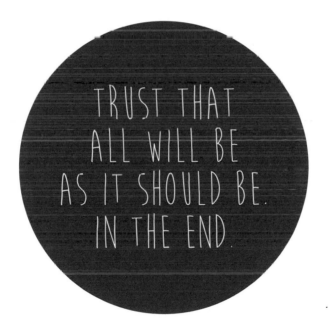

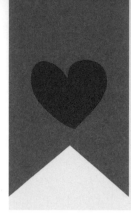

ON THIS DAY

DATE: _____

Fragrance is a powerful mood enhancer. Light a candle or inhale some essential oils.

MY NOTES
(WHAT I LOVED, FELT, WISHED, NEEDED, STRUGGLED WITH, OVERCAME)

....

....

....

....

....

....

....

....

....

....

....

TO DO LIST

❑ ....

❑ ....

❑ ....

❑ ....

❑ ....

THINGS TO REMEMBER
(BECAUSE A BABY ATE MY BRAIN)

....

....

....

....

....

MEMORIES TO RECALL
(YEARS FROM NOW)

....

....

....

....

....

BABY NOTES
(WHAT YOU DID, LOVED, NEEDED)

....

....

....

....

....

....

....

....

....

....

....

....

....

FEEDING NOTES
(TIME, DURATION/AMOUNT)

....

....

....

....

....

....

....

....

....

....

....

....

....

You are more resilient than ever. Because you now do far more on much less.

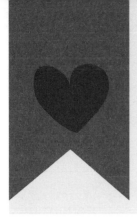

ON THIS DAY

DATE: _____

To your baby, there is no mum like you. You're their world.

MY NOTES
(WHAT I LOVED, FELT, WISHED, NEEDED, STRUGGLED WITH, OVERCAME)

....

....

....

....

....

....

....

TO DO LIST

....

- ☐ ....
- ☐ ....
- ☐ ....
- ☐ ....
- ☐ ....

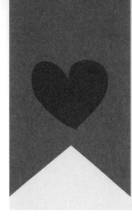

ON THIS DAY

DATE: _____

Give yourself permission to always feel how you're feeling. Whatever that is.

MY NOTES
(WHAT I LOVED, FELT, WISHED, NEEDED, STRUGGLED WITH, OVERCAME)

....

....

....

....

....

....

....

....

....

TO DO LIST

❑ ....

❑ ....

❑ ....

❑ ....

❑ ....

THINGS TO REMEMBER
(BECAUSE A BABY ATE MY BRAIN)

....

....

....

....

....

MEMORIES TO RECALL
(YEARS FROM NOW)

....

....

....

....

....

BABY NOTES
(WHAT YOU DID, LOVED, NEEDED)

....

....

....

....

....

....

....

....

....

....

....

....

....

FEEDING NOTES
(TIME, DURATION/AMOUNT)

....

....

....

....

....

....

....

....

....

....

....

....

....

FIVE MONTHS!

DID YOU EVER THINK YOU'D GET THIS FAR?

THREE WAYS I'VE EVOLVED:

1. ....

....

2. ....

....

3. ....

....

MONTH SIX

You are
good
enough.

'SHOULD I BE DOING BETTER?'

CHANGE CAN BE SCARY

As you approach the six-month mark, you're possibly feeling all nature of things. You might be wondering where the past six months have gone. You're maybe thinking about going back to work. You're starting to think about weaning your baby, or you've already begun.

A NEW MILESTONE

Reaching the six-month milestone can be quite emotional as your baby becomes more independent. You don't feel like such a new mum anymore. Sometimes you wonder if you're doing ok? Should you be doing better?

THE REALITY OF MOTHERHOOD

I've lost count of the number of times women have said to me, 'I'm not the mother I thought I'd be'. Myself included. But you know what? These preconceptions are exactly that… PRE-CONCEPTION. It's easy to say you'll be a patient, nurturing, tired-immune mother when you're sitting there, childless, in your skinny jeans with a glass of wine in your hand. The reality is a galaxy far, far away. Six months in, I'm sure you're already realising this.

YOU ARE GOOD ENOUGH

Asking yourself if you should be doing better is a question you'll never stop asking yourself as a mother. But there is only ever one answer and that is this: you are good enough. Because there is no one who could be better for your baby, your toddler, or your preschooler. Maybe in your (tired) eyes there is another mother out there doing 'better' than you. Who makes you question your efforts, or even your lack of effort because you're just too damn tired to make puree from scratch. Don't go there. Repeat, 'I am good enough.'

DON'T COMPARE YOURSELF

Who hasn't at one time or another felt rubbish at the hands of someone else? I know I have. But did THEY make us feel like that or did we do it to ourselves when we started to draw comparisons? Comparing yourself to another mum is a pointless habit because you're pitting yourself against a person that YOU perceive to be a certain way. A fictional character. That only exists in your mind. So next time you find yourself doing it, compare yourself to YOURSELF instead. Ask, 'How am I going to do better than I did yesterday?' Maybe you're not and that's ok too. But whatever you do, don't give away your energy focusing on anyone else but you and your baby.

NEVER JUDGE YOURSELF

The simple truth is your baby loves you, flaws and all. They don't judge you when you get it wrong. It's you who judges yourself and you need to stop. So, whenever you find yourself doubting yourself, comparing yourself to another mum or imagining that no one else is struggling like you feel you are, remember there isn't a mum in the land getting it right all of the time. Most of us are winging it, most of the time.

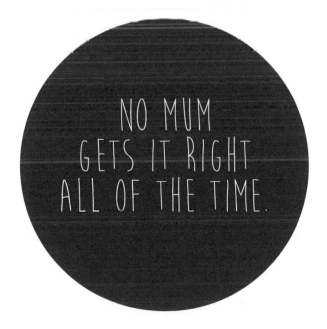

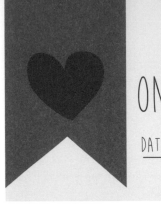

ON THIS DAY

DATE: _____

No mum is ever sure of herself. You're doing the best you can. Fact.

MY NOTES
(WHAT I LOVED, FELT, WISHED, NEEDED, STRUGGLED WITH, OVERCAME)

....

....

....

....

....

....

....

....

....

....

....

TO DO LIST

☐ ....

☐ ....

☐ ....

☐ ....

☐ ....

THINGS TO REMEMBER
(BECAUSE A BABY ATE MY BRAIN)

....

....

....

....

....

MEMORIES TO RECALL
(YEARS FROM NOW)

....

....

....

....

....

BABY NOTES
(WHAT YOU DID, LOVED, NEEDED)

....

....

....

....

....

....

....

....

....

....

....

....

....

WEANING NOTES
(WHAT YOU TRIED, LIKED, SPAT OUT)

....

....

....

....

....

....

....

....

....

....

....

....

....

There will be
GOOD days.
There will be
BAD days.

(you're not defined
by any of them.)

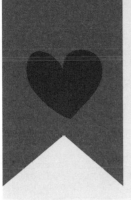

ON THIS DAY

DATE: _____

Give up on perfection. Embrace yourself like your baby does. With love.

MY NOTES
(WHAT I LOVED, FELT, WISHED, NEEDED, STRUGGLED WITH, OVERCAME)

....

....

....

....

....

....

....

....

....

....

....

TO DO LIST

☐ ....

☐ ....

☐ ....

☐ ....

☐ ....

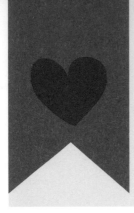

ON THIS DAY

DATE: _____

You don't realise your amazingness. But it's INSPIRING.

MY NOTES
(WHAT I LOVED, FELT, WISHED, NEEDED, STRUGGLED WITH, OVERCAME)

....

....

....

....

....

....

....

....

....

....

....

TO DO LIST

❏ ....

❏ ....

❏ ....

❏ ....

❏ ....

THINGS TO REMEMBER
(BECAUSE A BABY ATE MY BRAIN)

·······························

·······························

·······························

·······························

·······························

MEMORIES TO RECALL
(YEARS FROM NOW)

·······························

·······························

·······························

·······························

·······························

BABY NOTES
(WHAT YOU DID, LOVED, NEEDED)

·······························

·······························

·······························

·······························

·······························

·······························

·······························

·······························

·······························

·······························

·······························

·······························

·······························

WEANING NOTES
(WHAT YOU TRIED, LIKED, SPAT OUT)

·······························

·······························

·······························

·······························

·······························

·······························

·······························

·······························

·······························

·······························

·······························

·······························

·······························

I AM GOOD ENOUGH.

The End.

DATE: ....

SIGNED: ....

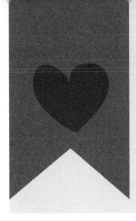

ON THIS DAY

DATE: _____

Routine up the wall? Don't stress. Go with the flow. Try again tomorrow.

MY NOTES
(WHAT I LOVED, FELT, WISHED, NEEDED, STRUGGLED WITH, OVERCAME)

....

....

....

....

....

....

....

TO DO LIST

❑ ....

❑ ....

❑ ....

❑ ....

❑ ....

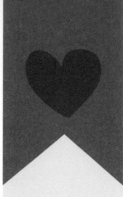

ON THIS DAY

DATE: _____

Feeling lonely?
Go out. It doesn't
matter where.
It only matters
that you do.

MY NOTES
(WHAT I LOVED, FELT, WISHED, NEEDED, STRUGGLED WITH, OVERCAME)

....

....

....

....

....

....

....

....

TO DO LIST

❏ ....

❏ ....

❏ ....

❏ ....

❏ ....

THINGS TO REMEMBER
(BECAUSE A BABY ATE MY BRAIN)

....

....

....

....

....

MEMORIES TO RECALL
(YEARS FROM NOW)

....

....

....

....

....

BABY NOTES
(WHAT YOU DID, LOVED, NEEDED)

....

....

....

....

....

....

....

....

....

....

....

....

....

....

WEANING NOTES
(WHAT YOU TRIED, LIKED, SPAT OUT)

....

....

....

....

....

....

....

....

....

....

....

....

....

HOW NOT TO WEAN YOUR BABY

Around the six-month mark you'll start to wean your baby. This is one of the first BIG milestones and a sign that your baby is growing up. Well, a little anyway. Weaning can feel overwhelming when you first begin. It's another thing to fit into your already busy life. But do you really have to puree every vegetable you come into contact with? Must you roast a chicken just to get the stock from it? You want to do it right, of course you do. You want to give your baby the best. But don't stress yourself out. Try and remember that popular parenting mantra, 'For the first year, FOOD IS FUN!' Oh yes. You'll be laughing your head off.

Here's a (light-hearted) look at what you need to know:

1. **Baby-led weaning or puree?** The main factor in making this decision is how you want to clean up food from the floor. Massacred florets of broccoli? Or pureed broccoli smeared into the kitchen tiles? Because regardless of how it goes in, that's where it all ends up. On the floor.

2. **Choose foods carefully.** Especially if your baby has a cold. Unless you enjoy being sneezed over with a mouthful of porridge. And let's face it, who doesn't enjoy that?

3. **Always wear a bib.** You. Not the baby. Because the food that doesn't end up on the floor? Ends up on you. (See above.)

4. **Sweet potato.** Do NOT feed this to your baby if you love it. Because after serving it every day and watching it come out the other end looking exactly the same as it went in, you won't want to touch it. Ever again. Superfood or not.

5. **Weaning kit.** Contrary to what experts, shops and catalogues will tell you, your baby WILL learn to eat without the following: 'special' weaning shaped bowls, 'special' weaning spoons and sterilising wipes. Very soon your crawling baby will be licking the floor and probably the cat's bowl. So why not save yourself some cash and just serve it in there to start with?

6. **Chicken stock.** You do NOT need to roast an Oxbridge-educated, caviar-fed, multi-lingual chicken just to get organic, low salt stock for your baby. Whilst this *is* a fun way to spend a Saturday night, it's exactly why low salt stock cubes were invented instead.

7. **Puree, glorious puree!** Likewise, you do not need to boil, puree and freeze every fruit and vegetable in the supermarket aisle. Not only will your baby decide they hate carrots but you'll then be forced to eat pureed carrot for the rest of time.

8. **Organic produce.** Whilst this may be the best start you can give your baby, ask yourself this: are you going to be feeding them crisps and party rings at their first birthday party? No? OK then, if you say so.

9. **Never give a baby chocolate.** This is a given, right? Except that unbeknown to you, your baby first tasted it shortly after birth when you left the room quickly to go for a poo and your friend's toddler shoved a chocolate finger in the baby's mouth.

10. **'Food is fun!'** You'll constantly be told that, for the first year, 'Food is fun!' Remember this. When your baby pukes REAL sick all over you. When they turn their nose up at the pureed chicken casserole you've spent six hours slow cooking. When they throw spinach puree at you in utter disgust. ALL OF THIS IS FUN. Got it?

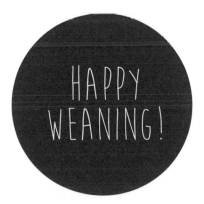

HAPPY WEANING!

ON THIS DAY

DATE: _____

It's ok to admit it's hard when the days stretch endlessly ahead.

MY NOTES
(WHAT I LOVED, FELT, WISHED, NEEDED, STRUGGLED WITH, OVERCAME)

....

....

....

....

....

....

....

....

....

....

TO DO LIST

❏ ....

❏ ....

❏ ....

❏ ....

❏ ....

THINGS TO REMEMBER
(BECAUSE A BABY ATE MY BRAIN)

·······································
·······································
·······································
·······································
·······································

MEMORIES TO RECALL
(YEARS FROM NOW)

·······································
·······································
·······································
·······································
·······································

BABY NOTES
(WHAT YOU DID, LOVED, NEEDED)

·······································
·······································
·······································
·······································
·······································
·······································
·······································
·······································
·······································
·······································
·······································
·······································
·······································

WEANING NOTES
(WHAT YOU TRIED, LIKED, SPAT OUT)

·······································
·······································
·······································
·······································
·······································
·······································
·······································
·······································
·······································
·······································
·······································
·······································
·······································

Whatever
happens
you're
going to be
just fine.

ON THIS DAY

DATE: _____

Got a smoothie maker? Blend any fruit and veg in the fridge for a pick-me-up.

MY NOTES
(WHAT I LOVED, FELT, WISHED, NEEDED, STRUGGLED WITH, OVERCAME)

....

....

....

....

....

....

TO DO LIST

- ☐ ....
- ☐ ....
- ☐ ....
- ☐ ....
- ☐ ....

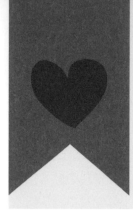

ON THIS DAY

DATE: _____

Some days, we're all just hanging on by a thread. And that's ok.

MY NOTES
(WHAT I LOVED, FELT, WISHED, NEEDED, STRUGGLED WITH, OVERCAME)

....

....

....

....

....

....

....

....

....

....

....

TO DO LIST

❑ ....

❑ ....

❑ ....

❑ ....

❑ ....

THINGS TO REMEMBER
(BECAUSE A BABY ATE MY BRAIN)

....

....

....

....

....

MEMORIES TO RECALL
(YEARS FROM NOW)

....

....

....

....

....

BABY NOTES
(WHAT YOU DID, LOVED, NEEDED)

....

....

....

....

....

....

....

....

....

....

....

....

....

WEANING NOTES
(WHAT YOU TRIED, LIKED, SPAT OUT)

....

....

....

....

....

....

....

....

....

....

....

....

....

THE NEW MUM F*CKET LIST

(8 THINGS YOU DO NOT NEED TO DO WHILST NURTURING A SMALL PERSON.)

You do NOT need to:

1. **Feel guilty about anything.** So what if you've been in your PJs for two days straight. So what if your older child is watching Netflix or the iPad all day. So what if no one's eaten anything more nutritious than a handful of raisins they found on the floor. The first three months (at least) are about SURVIVAL. Your survival and theirs. You do whatever you need to do to get through the day. Because when you have a small baby in tow, getting through the day is totally enough.

2. **Function.** In any way, shape or form. You do not need to be firing on all cylinders. You have nothing to prove. To yourself or the outside world. With baby number one, I remember going for a long walk three days after giving birth and feeling on top of the world, like I'd conquered it. 'A baby won't stop me!' I thought. On the way back, my stitches started to pull, I could barely get back up the hill and I felt like a bit of an idiot. The sofa is your best friend at the moment.

3. **Organise stuff.** When you're sitting around the house all day stuff preoccupies you. The chipped paint. The mess that occupies every dusty corner. The piles of junk you can never find a moment to sort. Forget it. Now is NOT the time to get busy.

4. **Do chores.** No one cares how messy your house is. If you haven't bleached your toilet for a week. If the washing up is still sitting on the side. YOU HAVE A SMALL BABY. The rest of the world can see this but when you're in a sleep-deprived fog, it's hard for you to see it yourself. You feel that it's a sign you're not coping. That you're not capable. It's not important, trust me. Get someone to help you with the chores. Hire a cleaner for the next couple of months if you're really that bothered. But let it go. You and your baby. That's what we care about.

5. **Justify yourself.** You are the most important person in the world right now. And anyone who doesn't get that by putting unfair expectations on you or pushing their own agendas can do one. You do what works for you and your family and you don't justify yourself to anyone. Got it?

6. **Question yourself.** None of us know what we're doing with a new baby. Don't worry about routines or feeding patterns or why your baby suddenly wants to eat ALL of the time. Just go with it for the first few months. You'll find it much easier to enjoy (tolerate) if you're not driving yourself mad with questions that are mostly impossible to answer.

7. **Diet.** I really hope this one is obvious but in case you're thinking about losing weight, don't. When you've had two hours sleep, cake is all you've got. Don't make yourself miserable going without the things you fancy. You've just done nine months of that, right?

8. **Go it alone.** Being a new mum can be lonely, no matter what round you're on. We haven't forgotten you, I promise. If we haven't checked in recently though and you're suddenly feeling overwhelmed, lonely or in need of some help, please ask. We'll be there in a heartbeat to do whatever we can do to get you through these early months. We know what it's like and we're right behind you. Keep going, you're doing brilliantly.

HALF A YEAR!

CUE NOSTALGIC THOUGHTS.
A FEW TEARS.
AND A DESIRE TO SLOW
THINGS DOWN.

HOW I WOULD SUM UP THE PAST SIX MONTHS:

....

....

....

....

....

....

MONTH SEVEN

The truth
about
relationships.

HOW PARENTHOOD CHANGES YOUR RELATIONSHIP

FOR BETTER FOR WORSE?

Before you had a baby, you probably imagined that having one would bring you and your partner closer together. Then this small, ever-so-demanding person came along and needed everything from you. Amidst the depths of tiredness and pure exhaustion it's completely normal to feel as if you're drifting apart. The early years of parenthood are tough on a relationship. Never underestimate that. You'll both feel the strain, in different ways. You might feel resentful that your partner seems to carry on much as they ever did. 'Nothing's really changed for them,' you think. 'Why don't they realise that this motherhood lark isn't all coffee and cakes? Why do they STILL not know where the nappies are kept?' Your other half likely has a very different perspective and is probably wondering why you suddenly seem so serious. So frazzled. And, some days, positively deranged. At odds with one another's lives, the cracks can start to appear.

FEELING UNAPPRECIATED

Most of the mothers I know, myself included, have at one time or another felt sheer disappointment at the hands of their partners. Why? Because, sometimes, we feel unappreciated. Misunderstood. And downright resentful. No one knows what motherhood really involves before they sign up. How tough it will be. How relentless. That it will mean giving up the right to a hot cup of tea, a moment's peace. That it will compromise our jobs, our bodies and our sanity. And mean working longer shifts than an A&E doctor. It's a selfless 'job' and it's always nice to have that acknowledged and be told, 'you're doing great'.

WHEN GETTING THE WORDS OUT IS HARD

Communication is one of the things that really suffers when you have a baby. You're tired and cranky. Your partner is also tired and may make thoughtless comments that make you angry. This combination means you're more likely to stare at the

TV in the evening than to want to try and talk to one another. Don't worry. This is really common amongst new parents. All parents, in fact. There are so many reasons that can make it difficult to connect.

MAKING TIME FOR ONE ANOTHER

It's the biggest cliché in the book. Making time for one another. Dare I mention the dreaded words, 'date night?' (Sorry.) The chances are that the thought of spending time together doesn't fill you with enthusiasm because you're knackered and also you might feel that you dislike one another a lot of the time. But getting away from your baby really helps to find some time and space to make that connection again. To remember that, actually, you do quite like each other. (If you don't want to leave your baby, have 'date night' at home. Just switch off TVs and phones!)

ASKING YOUR PARTNER TO PULL THEIR WEIGHT

Feeling valued is probably at the top of most mother's lists. You don't need to be worshipped or showered with gifts. You'd much rather just have a shower. In peace. Or given that oh so important acknowledgement and told that what you're doing is hard and you're doing amazingly. When the person you chose to have kids with realises that it's gestures like this (as well as putting out the bin and emptying the dishwasher) that make you feel valued? Then you start to feel like the team you always imagined you would be.

DRAW UP A ROTA

If your partner doesn't get this, even once you've told them, consider drawing up a rota for household chores. I know. You're not flatmates. But having something in writing can help. Lots of people function better with a list, to know where they stand and what's expected of them. And if it stops you sending them angry texts at work, well then everyone's a winner, right?

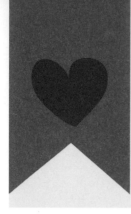

ON THIS DAY

DATE: _____

Raising a child is hard on your relationship. Never forget that.

MY NOTES
(WHAT I LOVED, FELT, WISHED, NEEDED, STRUGGLED WITH, OVERCAME)

....

....

....

....

....

....

....

....

....

....

....

TO DO LIST

❏ ....

❏ ....

❏ ....

❏ ....

❏ ....

THINGS TO REMEMBER
(BECAUSE A BABY ATE MY BRAIN)

....
....
....
....
....

MEMORIES TO RECALL
(YEARS FROM NOW)

....
....
....
....
....

BABY NOTES
(WHAT YOU DID, LOVED, NEEDED)

....
....
....
....
....
....
....
....
....
....
....
....
....

WEANING NOTES
(WHAT YOU TRIED, LIKED, SPAT OUT)

....
....
....
....
....
....
....
....
....
....
....
....
....

You deserve to hear
'YOU'RE AMAZING'
every single day.

(leave this page lying
around if you're not...)

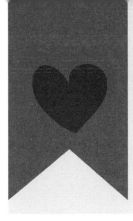

ON THIS DAY

DATE: _____

Tell your partner what you need from them. Don't leave them guessing.

MY NOTES
(WHAT I LOVED, FELT, WISHED, NEEDED, STRUGGLED WITH, OVERCAME)

....

....

....

....

....

....

....

....

....

....

....

TO DO LIST

❑ ....

❑ ....

❑ ....

❑ ....

❑ ....

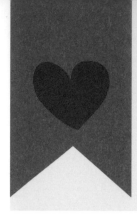

ON THIS DAY

DATE: _____

Ask your partner to be kind to you. Especially when you're cranky and tired.

MY NOTES
(WHAT I LOVED, FELT, WISHED, NEEDED, STRUGGLED WITH, OVERCAME)

....

....

....

....

....

....

....

....

....

....

....

TO DO LIST

❏ ....

❏ ....

❏ ....

❏ ....

❏ ....

THINGS TO REMEMBER
(BECAUSE A BABY ATE MY BRAIN)

....

....

....

....

....

MEMORIES TO RECALL
(YEARS FROM NOW)

....

....

....

....

....

BABY NOTES
(WHAT YOU DID, LOVED, NEEDED)

....

....

....

....

....

....

....

....

....

....

....

....

....

....

WEANING NOTES
(WHAT YOU TRIED, LIKED, SPAT OUT)

....

....

....

....

....

....

....

....

....

....

....

....

....

Things I would like from my partner...

(this may be practical help with chores or some emotional support.)

- ☐ ....
  ....

- ☐ ....
  ....

- ☐ ....
  ....

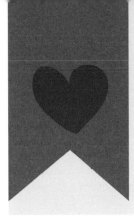

ON THIS DAY

DATE:

Set a night(s) for your partner to cook dinner.

MY NOTES
(WHAT I LOVED, FELT, WISHED, NEEDED, STRUGGLED WITH, OVERCAME)

....

....

....

....

....

....

....

....

....

....

....

TO DO LIST

❏ ....

❏ ....

❏ ....

❏ ....

❏ ....

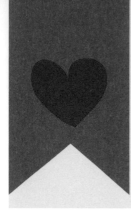

ON THIS DAY

DATE: _____

If you can't remember when you and your partner had an hour together, it's time to find one.

MY NOTES
(WHAT I LOVED, FELT, WISHED, NEEDED, STRUGGLED WITH, OVERCAME)

....

....

....

....

....

....

....

....

....

....

....

TO DO LIST

❑ ....

❑ ....

❑ ....

❑ ....

❑ ....

THINGS TO REMEMBER
(BECAUSE A BABY ATE MY BRAIN)

....

....

....

....

....

MEMORIES TO RECALL
(YEARS FROM NOW)

....

....

....

....

....

BABY NOTES
(WHAT YOU DID, LOVED, NEEDED)

....

....

....

....

....

....

....

....

....

....

....

....

....

WEANING NOTES
(WHAT YOU TRIED, LIKED, SPAT OUT)

....

....

....

....

....

....

....

....

....

....

....

....

....

HOUSEHOLD ROTA

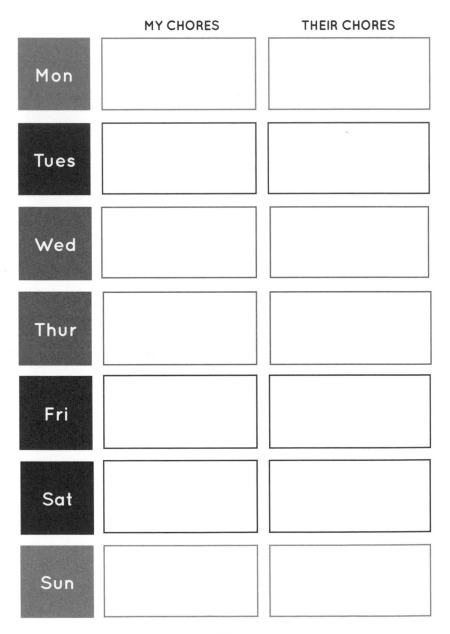

	MY CHORES	THEIR CHORES
Mon		
Tues		
Wed		
Thur		
Fri		
Sat		
Sun		

DATE NIGHT
SPICY SAUSAGE PASTA

This is a really easy dish for your other half to prepare for you. It's filling, has a bit of a kick to it and the combination of the sausage, feta and coriander is lush. You can substitute/omit/adjust any ingredients, as you prefer. Serve with garlic bread, a rocket salad and a glass of red. Follow with a couple of (shop bought) melting middle chocolate puddings. And turn off the TV.

INGREDIENTS (eat 2, freeze 2 without pasta)

6 good quality sausages, skins removed

Olive oil

1 onion, chopped

4 tablespoons of pitted black olives, quartered

3 tablespoons of capers

$\frac{1}{2}$ teaspoon of chilli flakes

500g passata

200g rigatoni pasta

100g feta cheese

2 good handfuls of fresh coriander, chopped

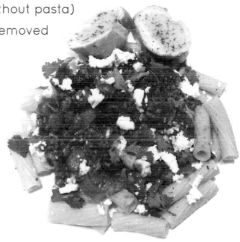

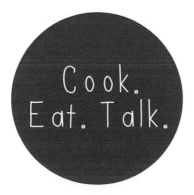

Cook.
Eat. Talk.

METHOD

Fry the onions in the oil. Mince the sausage meat with a fork and add to onions, stirring until browned. Add the passata, olives, capers and chilli flakes. Simmer for 20 minutes. Cook the pasta. Serve the sauce on top with a good handful of feta and coriander.

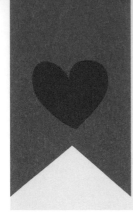

ON THIS DAY

DATE:

Do something nice for one another. Or say something nice.

MY NOTES
(WHAT I LOVED, FELT, WISHED, NEEDED, STRUGGLED WITH, OVERCAME)

....

....

....

....

....

....

TO DO LIST

.... ❏ ....

.... ❏ ....

.... ❏ ....

.... ❏ ....

.... ❏ ....

THINGS TO REMEMBER
(BECAUSE A BABY ATE MY BRAIN)

....
....
....
....
....

MEMORIES TO RECALL
(YEARS FROM NOW)

....
....
....
....
....

BABY NOTES
(WHAT YOU DID, LOVED, NEEDED)

....
....
....
....
....
....
....
....
....
....
....
....
....
....

WEANING NOTES
(WHAT YOU TRIED, LIKED, SPAT OUT)

....
....
....
....
....
....
....
....
....
....
....
....
....
....

Understanding
what you both
need is the key
to being a team.
TELL EACH OTHER.

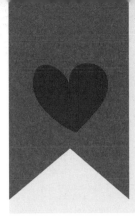

ON THIS DAY

DATE: _____

It's easy to focus on flaws. Think of something your partner does that makes you smile.

MY NOTES
(WHAT I LOVED, FELT, WISHED, NEEDED, STRUGGLED WITH, OVERCAME)

....

....

....

....

....

....

....

....

....

....

....

....

TO DO LIST

❏ ....

❏ ....

❏ ....

❏ ....

❏ ....

ON THIS DAY

DATE: _____

If you'd like flowers, drop hints. If that doesn't work, treat yourself to a bunch.

MY NOTES
(WHAT I LOVED, FELT, WISHED, NEEDED, STRUGGLED WITH, OVERCAME)

....

....

....

....

....

....

....

....

TO DO LIST

- ❏ ....
- ❏ ....
- ❏ ....
- ❏ ....
- ❏ ....

THINGS TO REMEMBER
(BECAUSE A BABY ATE MY BRAIN)

....
....
....
....
....

MEMORIES TO RECALL
(YEARS FROM NOW)

....
....
....
....
....

BABY NOTES
(WHAT YOU DID, LOVED, NEEDED)

....
....
....
....
....
....
....
....
....
....
....
....
....

WEANING NOTES
(WHAT YOU TRIED, LIKED, SPAT OUT)

....
....
....
....
....
....
....
....
....
....
....
....
....

SEVEN MONTHS!

HOWEVER HARD THINGS FEEL SOMETIMES, JUST LOOK HOW HAPPY YOUR BABY IS.

(YOU'RE DOING THAT.)

THREE THINGS WE COULD WORK ON:

1. ....
   ....

2. ....
   ....

3. ....
   ....

MONTH EIGHT

Are you feeling lonely?

A LETTER TO A LONELY MUM

Dear Lonely Mum,

I'm writing to say hello. To see how you're doing. To let you know that I KNOW. I know what it feels like to be lonely. To find this motherhood lark isolating and confusing. To wonder if you've made a horrible mistake and if you'll ever feel like yourself again. To love your baby but still to want to press the rewind button.

I write now because today I have a few more answers than I did yesterday. And I want to share them with you. So you can perhaps feel a little less lonely tomorrow. So you can tap into the courage that is already there, deep in the pit of your stomach beneath all the butterflies and the sinking feeling that pops up out of nowhere. And stops you in your tracks.

Would you believe me if I said you're not the only one who feels like this? That all mums feel this sense of loneliness regardless of how popular they are? I've had three babies. And, now I look back, loneliness has been there each time, waiting in the wings. To trip me up. Play tricks on me. And knock my confidence.

It wasn't that I didn't have friends. It was just that looking after a baby, then a baby and a toddler, then a baby, a preschooler and a schooler was sometimes so relentless that I didn't have the time or the energy to connect with those around me. All my energies were needed elsewhere. Some days there was nothing left for me. I had nothing more to give. Loneliness preys on that in order to survive.

You know this first-hand, I know. There are days where you don't see another adult between the hours of 7.00 AM and 7.00 PM. Where your only company is the sound of your baby crying. Or are those tears coming from you? Those days are tough. They cripple you. They stop you from being part of the outside world. A world it seems you long since left. A world that carries on without you and cruelly shuts you out. Because when you have a baby, everything changes.

Suddenly, everything you did so easily and without thought, that you took for granted, now takes effort and consideration. You can't leave the house without a three-pronged attack. Can you be bothered? Maybe you'll just stay in.

But don't stay in. Please don't. I know you're tired and you don't have anywhere in particular to go. But that world is still there. It doesn't matter where you go. It only matters that you do. To the park. For a coffee. Chat to the barista. Strike up a conversation with that other mum in the park. A mum who is probably in the park for the same reason that you are. Because she feels a bit lonely. A bit lost. It will feel awkward. You will question what you'll get out of it, really. You already have enough friends, you don't need any more. But you know what? You do need more. At this stage in your life you need other mum friends. People like you. You need people that live locally to you, so you feel connected. So it's easy to meet up. So you feel part of something.

If you can face it, go somewhere where you know there'll be other mums. A baby class. Or a playgroup. It will feel strange to start with. Forced even. And like everyone knows one another. But they are probably all going through the motions, just as you are. Feeling as uncomfortable. And if it turns out that everyone does know each other, remember this: they once stood where you stand now. I once stood where you stand now. I'd never been to a playgroup until baby number three. Imagine! But then it saved my soul. Having a regular place to go is so important. But having a cup of tea made for you? A fleeting chat with someone who just gets it? You can't put a value on that.

I've heard mums say that the playgroup they went to was cliquey. I'm so sorry when that happens, but often it's just because they are busy places. So don't go away feeling all your effort was wasted. Go back next week. Speak to someone. Anyone. Because that mum you talked to? They'll be so glad you did. You made a difference to their day. You made them feel less alone. YOU. Who almost didn't leave the house this morning. How amazing are you?

Sending love and understanding (and a huge slice of cake).

Amy x

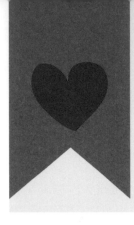

ON THIS DAY

DATE: _____

There's no shame in feeling lonely. We've all been there.

MY NOTES
(WHAT I LOVED, FELT, WISHED, NEEDED, STRUGGLED WITH, OVERCAME)

....

....

....

....

....

....

....

....

....

....

....

TO DO LIST

❏ ....

❏ ....

❏ ....

❏ ....

❏ ....

THINGS TO REMEMBER
(BECAUSE A BABY ATE MY BRAIN)

....

....

....

....

....

MEMORIES TO RECALL
(YEARS FROM NOW)

....

....

....

....

....

BABY NOTES
(WHAT YOU DID, LOVED, NEEDED)

....

....

....

....

....

....

....

....

....

....

....

....

....

WEANING NOTES
(WHAT YOU TRIED, LIKED, SPAT OUT)

....

....

....

....

....

....

....

....

....

....

....

....

Go out.
It doesn't matter
where you go. It
only matters that
you do.

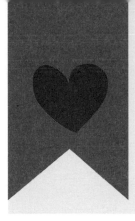

ON THIS DAY

DATE: _____

Talk to another mum. She's probably feeling the same as you are.

MY NOTES
(WHAT I LOVED, FELT, WISHED, NEEDED, STRUGGLED WITH, OVERCAME)

....

....

....

....

....

....

....

....

....

....

....

TO DO LIST

❏ ....

❏ ....

❏ ....

❏ ....

❏ ....

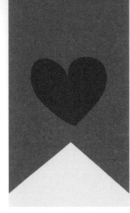

ON THIS DAY

DATE: _____

Finding it hard to meet other mums? Try a 'mummy social' app.

MY NOTES
(WHAT I LOVED, FELT, WISHED, NEEDED, STRUGGLED WITH, OVERCAME)

....

....

....

....

....

....

....

....

....

....

....

TO DO LIST

☐ ....

☐ ....

☐ ....

☐ ....

☐ ....

THINGS TO REMEMBER
(BECAUSE A BABY ATE MY BRAIN)

....

....

....

....

....

MEMORIES TO RECALL
(YEARS FROM NOW)

....

....

....

....

....

BABY NOTES
(WHAT YOU DID, LOVED, NEEDED)

....

....

....

....

....

....

....

....

....

....

....

....

....

WEANING NOTES
(WHAT YOU TRIED, LIKED, SPAT OUT)

....

....

....

....

....

....

....

....

....

....

....

....

....

Things I can do/ places I can go to feel less lonely.

(add details of regular playgroups, baby classes, drop in centres.)

MONDAY ....

TUESDAY ....

WEDNESDAY ....

THURSDAY ....

FRIDAY ....

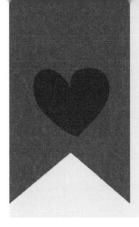

ON THIS DAY

DATE: _____

Don't let loneliness knock your confidence. You're still the same, wonderful YOU.

MY NOTES
(WHAT I LOVED, FELT, WISHED, NEEDED, STRUGGLED WITH, OVERCAME)

....

....

....

....

....

....

....

....

....

....

....

TO DO LIST

❏ ....

❏ ....

❏ ....

❏ ....

❏ ....

ON THIS DAY

DATE: _____

Tough days can cripple you. Do something that lifts your mood.

MY NOTES
(WHAT I LOVED, FELT, WISHED, NEEDED, STRUGGLED WITH, OVERCAME)

....

....

....

....

....

....

....

....

....

TO DO LIST

❑ ....

❑ ....

❑ ....

❑ ....

❑ ....

THINGS TO REMEMBER
(BECAUSE A BABY ATE MY BRAIN)

....
....
....
....
....

MEMORIES TO RECALL
(YEARS FROM NOW)

....
....
....
....
....

BABY NOTES
(WHAT YOU DID, LOVED, NEEDED)

....
....
....
....
....
....
....
....
....
....
....
....
....

WEANING NOTES
(WHAT YOU TRIED, LIKED, SPAT OUT)

....
....
....
....
....
....
....
....
....
....
....
....
....

LOTS OF MUMS FEEL ANXIOUS

WHEN THOUGHTS BECOME SCARY

One of the side effects of loneliness is having too much time to think and breeding thoughts that have the freedom to run wild. One of the things lots of new mums have mentioned is feeling anxious. About things that never made them feel anxious before, especially their own mortality. It's a frightening realisation and one that can quickly consume you, if you let it.

IT'S NORMAL

I'm sure if someone was to research this, they would find that there is a syndrome which plagues mothers of new babies and young children. A syndrome which makes them worry about dying and leaving their offspring when they need their mothers most. Something that is scary but is also actually a deep-seated, natural reaction to the responsibility that comes with having someone completely dependent upon you. Something that is made worse by how tired, stretched and claustrophobic you sometimes feel. But something that is completely normal.

'WHY NOT ME?'

I have experienced health anxiety after the birth of each of my children. I've had all sorts of strange physical symptoms as a result and gone to bed at night worrying that I won't wake up. And wondering what will happen to my children if I'm not around (aside from the obvious things like their dad dressing them in tights and sandals and letting them eat chocolate cereal and baked beans until the end of time). This type of health anxiety, which is so common in new mums, can be triggered by any variety of things and is often exacerbated by the world we live in. The world that shares everything via social networking platforms like Facebook and Twitter. The world that makes you think, 'Why NOT me next?' The world that no longer allows you to live in blissful ignorance.

IT'S ALL RELATIVE

These days, our Facebook and Twitter feeds tell us about things we would never otherwise know about. We hear about the hardships and tragedies that befall strangers (including our peers, those mothers of children that are so like us), living hundreds of miles away, when 30 years ago we'd have only known about those living at the end of our road. Suddenly, the odds don't seem to be in our favour, when in reality it is much more likely to be a case of our social reach being wider. And us knowing more than perhaps is good for us.

GET IT INTO PERSPECTIVE

It's important to remember all of this. To sometimes get it into perspective. These feelings of anxiety are commonly felt and nothing to be ashamed of. They're better once shared, so speak to another mum. These feelings don't make you less intelligent, capable or funny. They make you more real and connected with others. Because at 3.00AM it helps to know that somewhere, not so far away, another mum is lying awake worrying about the things that you are worrying about. Like whether their other half can do a plait. Or knows that a potato is not actually one of your five a day. You're not crazy. And you're definitely not alone. You're a mum, who wants the best for your child.

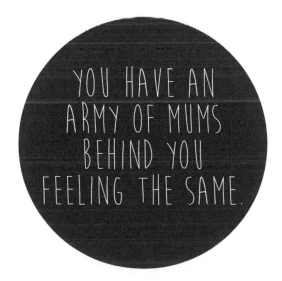

181

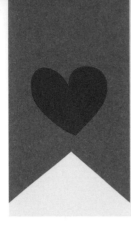

ON THIS DAY

DATE: _____

If you're feeling vulnerable, switch off social media. And breathe.

MY NOTES
(WHAT I LOVED, FELT, WISHED, NEEDED, STRUGGLED WITH, OVERCAME)

....

....

....

....

....

....

....

TO DO LIST

❏ ....

❏ ....

❏ ....

❏ ....

❏ ....

THINGS TO REMEMBER
(BECAUSE A BABY ATE MY BRAIN)

....

....

....

....

....

MEMORIES TO RECALL
(YEARS FROM NOW)

....

....

....

....

....

BABY NOTES
(WHAT YOU DID, LOVED, NEEDED)

....

....

....

....

....

....

....

....

....

....

....

....

....

WEANING NOTES
(WHAT YOU TRIED, LIKED, SPAT OUT)

....

....

....

....

....

....

....

....

....

....

....

....

....

ALL MUMS
FEEL ANXIOUS
AT ONE TIME OR
ANOTHER.

(you're not going crazy.)

ON THIS DAY

DATE: _____

Don't let anxious thoughts become catastrophic. Get back in the 'now'.

MY NOTES
(WHAT I LOVED, FELT, WISHED, NEEDED, STRUGGLED WITH, OVERCAME)

....

....

....

....

....

....

....

....

....

....

....

TO DO LIST

❏ ....

❏ ....

❏ ....

❏ ....

❏ ....

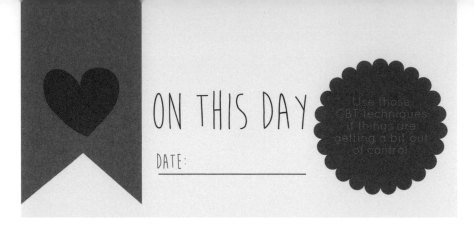

ON THIS DAY

DATE: _____

Use those CBT techniques if things are getting a bit out of control.

MY NOTES
(WHAT I LOVED, FELT, WISHED, NEEDED, STRUGGLED WITH, OVERCAME)

....

....

....

....

....

....

....

....

....

....

....

TO DO LIST

☐ ....

☐ ....

☐ ....

☐ ....

☐ ....

THINGS TO REMEMBER
(BECAUSE A BABY ATE MY BRAIN)

....

....

....

....

....

MEMORIES TO RECALL
(YEARS FROM NOW)

....

....

....

....

....

BABY NOTES
(WHAT YOU DID, LOVED, NEEDED)

....

....

....

....

....

....

....

....

....

....

....

....

....

WEANING NOTES
(WHAT YOU TRIED, LIKED, SPAT OUT)

....

....

....

....

....

....

....

....

....

....

....

....

....

EIGHT MONTHS!
IT'S QUITE REMARKABLE HOW WELL YOU'RE DOING.

(GIVE YOURSELF A BIG PAT ON THE BACK.)

THREE WAYS I'VE FELT MORE CONNECTED:

1. ....

....

2. ....

....

3. ....

....

MONTH NINE

Ditch
the
guilt.

ALL MUMS FEEL GUILTY

A MOTHER'S PREROGATIVE

No one tells you that when you give birth you'll not only get a baby, but also a lifetime supply of guilt. An emotion that can rear its head regardless of whether things are going well or not. And one that all mums have to learn to live with. They don't tell you this on the NCT course – that guilt is a mother's prerogative. I guess it's not a strong selling point. 'Come to NCT. Let us tell you about the joys of motherhood. How to rock labour on just a glass of wine. Oh and meet Guilt, your new other half.'

THERE'S ALWAYS SOMETHING TO FEEL GUILTY ABOUT

Feeling guilty is something that most of us suffer from once we become mothers. In the early months, you might feel guilty about any number of things, from how you're feeding your baby to how you're getting them to sleep to sometimes feeling a bit resentful of this little person who has changed the way you see yourself. As your baby grows, so does the guilt. You might feel guilty that you aren't playing with them enough. You might feel guilty if you're leaving them to go back to work. You may even feel guilty if you *don't* feel guilty about leaving them (because you secretly quite enjoy the break). The list is endless.

CAN YOU WIN?

Yes. And no. Lives are complex these days. You want to be a good mother, whilst possibly having a career, running a home and also wanting space to be yourself. But there is never enough time so you end up feeling permanently guilty about whatever you're not doing in any given moment. But you can't do it all. Not well, anyway. Or in a fulfilling manner. Multi-tasking is about as big a myth as saying, 'You can have it all'. You can't, so stop trying. Get back to the moment that's happening now and shelve those guilty, unhelpful thoughts.

THE MYTH OF MOTHERHOOD

A lot of the guilt we feel comes from the misconception that this motherhood lark should come naturally. We're led to believe that mothering is the most natural thing in the world. So when it doesn't feel like that, or we have periods where we're struggling, we feel like freaks of nature. And we feel guilty that we aren't better at the one thing we were apparently born to do. Rest assured: becoming a mother *may* be natural, but it's also relentless. Challenging. And overwhelming. When your baby is young, it feels like it will never, ever get easier. Don't feel guilty if you ever have these feelings. If you're wishing the day, or the week, away. Saying the words out loud can help. Because when we share our perceived inadequacies with one another and are honest about just how hard it is, we feel better. The relief is palpable. Of course, in low moments, it's easy to forget this and imagine that everyone else is doing a better job than you. But they're not. We're all just flying by the seat of our big, comfy pants. I promise you.

TO THE MOON AND BACK

If you just can't ditch the guilt, don't feel guilty about *that*. Because actually? It *is* OK to feel guilty. If you think about it, the guilt you feel as a mother comes from loving your child to the moon and back. From your desire to do right by them. To be the best mother that you can be and to give them as much of you as they deserve. So, next time you feel that pang of guilt, instead of berating yourself, stop for a moment and acknowledge it for what it really is. Love. Complete and utter unconditional love. You're doing the best you can. And it *is* good enough.

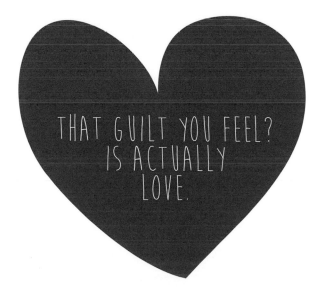

THAT GUILT YOU FEEL?
IS ACTUALLY
LOVE.

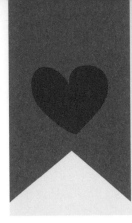

ON THIS DAY

DATE:

Why do you think you need to be better? You're already BRILLIANT.

MY NOTES
(WHAT I LOVED, FELT, WISHED, NEEDED, STRUGGLED WITH, OVERCAME)

....

....

....

....

....

....

....

....

....

....

....

TO DO LIST

❑ ....

❑ ....

❑ ....

❑ ....

❑ ....

THINGS TO REMEMBER
(BECAUSE A BABY ATE MY BRAIN)

....
....
....
....
....

MEMORIES TO RECALL
(YEARS FROM NOW)

....
....
....
....
....

BABY NOTES
(WHAT YOU DID, LOVED, NEEDED)

....
....
....
....
....
....
....
....
....
....
....
....
....

WEANING NOTES
(WHAT YOU TRIED, LIKED, SPAT OUT)

....
....
....
....
....
....
....
....
....
....
....
....
....

Being the perfect
mother is a myth.
Being an imperfect
one is a gift.

(because you show your child
it's ok to be human.)

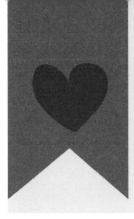

ON THIS DAY

DATE: _____

You'll never get it right ALL of the time. So stop trying. And accept yourself.

MY NOTES
(WHAT I LOVED, FELT, WISHED, NEEDED, STRUGGLED WITH, OVERCAME)

....

....

....

....

....

....

....

....

....

....

....

TO DO LIST

❑ ....

❑ ....

❑ ....

❑ ....

❑ ....

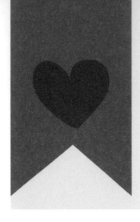

ON THIS DAY

DATE: _____

A lot of guilt comes from unrealistic expectations. Lower them.

MY NOTES
(WHAT I LOVED, FELT, WISHED, NEEDED, STRUGGLED WITH, OVERCAME)

....

....

....

....

....

....

....

TO DO LIST

❏ ....

❏ ....

❏ ....

❏ ....

❏ ....

THINGS TO REMEMBER
(BECAUSE A BABY ATE MY BRAIN)

....
....
....
....
....

MEMORIES TO RECALL
(YEARS FROM NOW)

....
....
....
....
....

BABY NOTES
(WHAT YOU DID, LOVED, NEEDED)

....
....
....
....
....
....
....
....
....
....
....
....
....

WEANING NOTES
(WHAT YOU TRIED, LIKED, SPAT OUT)

....
....
....
....
....
....
....
....
....
....
....
....
....

What did you do RIGHT today?

(write down something you did WELL.)

....

....

....

....

....

....

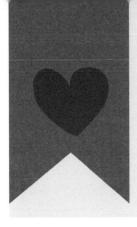

ON THIS DAY

DATE: _____

You're always doing the best by your baby. How can that ever be wrong?

MY NOTES
(WHAT I LOVED, FELT, WISHED, NEEDED, STRUGGLED WITH, OVERCAME)

....

....

....

....

....

....

....

....

....

....

TO DO LIST

☐ ....

☐ ....

☐ ....

☐ ....

☐ ....

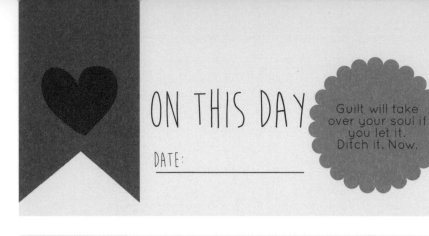

ON THIS DAY

Guilt will take over your soul if you let it. Ditch it. Now.

DATE: _____

MY NOTES
(WHAT I LOVED, FELT, WISHED, NEEDED, STRUGGLED WITH, OVERCAME)

....

....

....

....

....

....

....

....

....

....

....

TO DO LIST

☐ ....

☐ ....

☐ ....

☐ ....

☐ ....

THINGS TO REMEMBER
(BECAUSE A BABY ATE MY BRAIN)

....

....

....

....

....

MEMORIES TO RECALL
(YEARS FROM NOW)

....

....

....

....

....

BABY NOTES
(WHAT YOU DID, LOVED, NEEDED)

....

....

....

....

....

....

....

....

....

....

....

....

....

WEANING NOTES
(WHAT YOU TRIED, LIKED, SPAT OUT)

....

....

....

....

....

....

....

....

....

....

....

....

....

WHAT DID YOU DO RIGHT TODAY?

CUT YOURSELF SOME SLACK

When we become mums, as well as feeling guilty we also develop the habit of focusing on all the stuff we do badly. Losing our tempers. Losing our patience. Losing our keys. What happened to cutting ourselves some slack and recognising all the things we do WELL?

'OH, IT'S SUCH A PERFECT DAY'

Since having children, I have had to let go of any aspirations of the perfect day. I'm not sure it really existed before. It certainly doesn't exist now. But I still mourn it. And at the end of the day I have a tendency to berate myself if I lost my temper or screamed at the kids or just wasn't as perfect a mother as I could have been. Because at the back of my mind there is this alter ego of a mother. She is always kind. Always patient and understanding. She handles tantrums with a smile. AND she does crafts.

YOU DON'T NEED TO BE PERFECT

I blame Julie Andrews for this mental image. She should have done a follow-up movie called *Mary Crappins*. Where Mary has her own kids, realises what actual hell it is and hits the booze. Hard. Because quite frankly, there is too much pressure on women today to be the perfect mother. 'Protect your children. From absolutely everything. Whilst being brilliant and composed. All of the time.' It can leave us feeling overcautious, overwhelmed and that we will literally be scarring our children forever with every wrong turn we make.

BEING IMPERFECT IS A GIFT

But wrong turns are par for the course. And there's nothing 'wrong' with them, especially if you go back and try and make the right turn. Because our children learn from our mistakes. They learn from our reactions. They learn that it is ok to be human. And that they don't have to live up to an ideal of perfection that is impossible to maintain. Or, worse, live in fear of disappointing us.

S*** HAPPENS

I remember one occasion where I was upset in front of my eldest daughter. Now, my alter ego would have waited until her children were in bed to exhibit any signs of sadness. Even then she probably would have sobbed quietly into a tissue before giving herself a good talking to and pulling herself together. But in real life things happen. Suddenly and without warning. And it isn't always possible to compose yourself and deal with the fall-out later. Did she feel frightened? Did she feel insecure? No. With utter confidence she put her arm around me and with a soothing voice she said, 'Mummy, I know what will make you feel better. Get into bed with me and we'll read your favourite story together.' It wasn't my finest hour but it was definitely hers.

YOU'RE ONLY HUMAN

When I retold this to my friend, I focused on all the negatives of the situation. How I shouldn't have cried in front of my daughter. How she shouldn't be the one comforting me. How I should be a better mother. 'Where do you think she learned that behaviour?' said my friend. 'Where do you think she learned to nurture and care for another human being? From you. That doesn't make you a bad mother. It makes you a great one.' And yet, it hadn't even occurred to me to think of it like that.

BE KIND TO YOURSELF

Sometimes we're not very kind to ourselves. Most of us wouldn't treat another person the way we often treat ourselves. So take a vow. To be kind. To yourself. Don't waste your energy focusing on all the many things you could do better as a mother. Instead look at what you've done well in any given day. Because there is always something. Yes, you might have to look for it. Because the positives have the misfortune of sometimes getting lost under the negatives that are always so much easier to see. But look and you shall find. And at the end of each day, rather than dwelling on all the things you think you did wrong, ask yourself this instead: 'What did I do RIGHT today?'

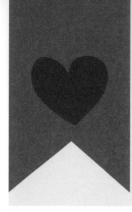

ON THIS DAY

DATE: _____

Feeling guilty uses up energy. You could do something WONDERFUL with that energy instead.

MY NOTES
(WHAT I LOVED, FELT, WISHED, NEEDED, STRUGGLED WITH, OVERCAME)

....

....

....

....

....

....

....

TO DO LIST

.... ❑ ....

.... ❑ ....

.... ❑ ....

.... ❑ ....

.... ❑ ....

THINGS TO REMEMBER
(BECAUSE A BABY ATE MY BRAIN)

....

....

....

....

....

MEMORIES TO RECALL
(YEARS FROM NOW)

....

....

....

....

....

BABY NOTES
(WHAT YOU DID, LOVED, NEEDED)

....

....

....

....

....

....

....

....

....

....

....

....

WEANING NOTES
(WHAT YOU TRIED, LIKED, SPAT OUT)

....

....

....

....

....

....

....

....

....

....

....

....

No one's the mother they THOUGHT they'd be. But you ARE the mother you're meant to be.

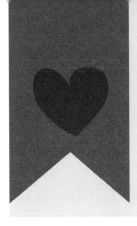

ON THIS DAY

DATE: _____

Think happy thoughts. It's hard to feel guilty when you're smiling.

MY NOTES
(WHAT I LOVED, FELT, WISHED, NEEDED, STRUGGLED WITH, OVERCAME)

....

....

....

....

....

....

....

TO DO LIST

❑ ....

❑ ....

....

❑ ....

....

❑ ....

....

❑ ....

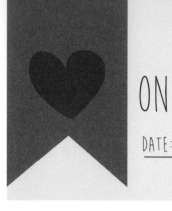

ON THIS DAY

DATE: _____

You can never win at a game where the rules are always changing. Just keep going.

MY NOTES
(WHAT I LOVED, FELT, WISHED, NEEDED, STRUGGLED WITH, OVERCAME)

....

....

....

....

....

....

....

....

....

....

....

TO DO LIST

❑ ....

❑ ....

❑ ....

❑ ....

❑ ....

THINGS TO REMEMBER
(BECAUSE A BABY ATE MY BRAIN)

....
....
....
....
....

MEMORIES TO RECALL
(YEARS FROM NOW)

....
....
....
....
....

BABY NOTES
(WHAT YOU DID, LOVED, NEEDED)

....
....
....
....
....
....
....
....
....
....
....
....

WEANING NOTES
(WHAT YOU TRIED, LIKED, SPAT OUT)

....
....
....
....
....
....
....
....
....
....
....
....

NINE MONTHS!

YOU ARE THE PERFECT MOTHER FOR YOUR BABY.

THREE WAYS I'VE LEARNED TO DITCH THE GUILT:

1. ....

....

2. ....

....

3. ....

....

MONTH TEN

Find
your mum
mojo.

THE SECRET OF MUM MOJO

'WHO AM I?'

There's a lot of talk about 'losing your identity' when you become a mum. In fact, I think it's such a buzz phrase these days, we're all petrified that one day we're simply going to evaporate. So we spend our days running around trying to find ourselves whilst feeding a baby and sticking the washing on. But becoming a mum doesn't mean we have to lose our identity. In fact, I think it can actually help us find it. Suddenly, we understand unconditional love. We understand real priorities. We understand just how much we are capable of. It gives us our 'mum mojo'. That enables us to do anything we put our minds to.

'WHAT'S MUM MOJO?'

Basically? It's your awesomeness. Your inner resourcefulness. Your ability to reach the brink, bounce back and be even more amazing than you were yesterday.

'HAVE I GOT IT?'

Yes! Every mum has it in abundance. The strength mums possess is amazing. Both emotionally and physically. We push babies in buggies whilst carrying bags and a tantruming toddler. We negotiate everything most days to get our kids to do anything. We fight little battles every day. And I think us mums might just be the strongest force in the world. Our patience. Our agility. Our sheer determination. No one trains us. We don't get time to be as fit as we'd like to be. We withstand all sorts of 'torture' like sleep deprivation and psychological mind games. And yet we keep going. Somehow. We find the inner strength to survive another day. And face the next one with a smile. *That* is mum mojo. And you have *plenty* of it.

ROCK YOUR MUM MOJO

Motherhood can be an amazing source of inspiration. There's something about having babies that makes women more creative. It helps us look at the world around us with fresh eyes. And it broadens our social circle and puts us amongst women we might not have the opportunity to meet if we didn't have motherhood in common. This is a real gift because we learn from newness and connecting with others. We can be invigorated and inspired by it. And it can lead us to do things we never even imagined we could do.

IGNITE YOUR PASSION

The desire to use our minds again or find a way to work flexibly around our families can lead to all sorts of wonderful ideas, many of which turn into actual businesses. There are mums out there making real livings out of their experiences and passions. Would you like that to be you? Talk to other mums who inspire you, for whatever reason. Write down any ideas you have, no matter how far fetched they may seem. Finally, take your time, there's no rush. Anything is possible. Because you are YOU.

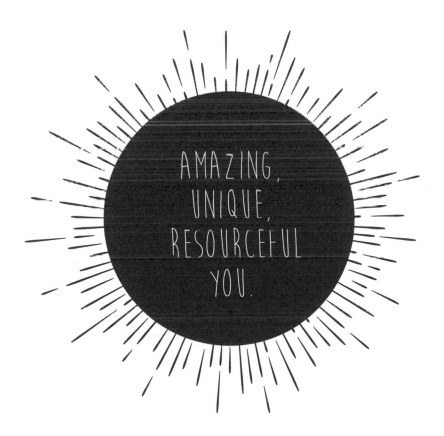

AMAZING,
UNIQUE,
RESOURCEFUL
YOU.

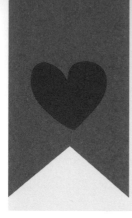

ON THIS DAY

DATE: _____

Use this time
to do the things
you hoped you'd
do on maternity.
That art gallery?
Go!

MY NOTES
(WHAT I LOVED, FELT, WISHED, NEEDED, STRUGGLED WITH, OVERCAME)

....

....

....

....

....

....

....

....

....

....

....

TO DO LIST

❑ ....

❑ ....

❑ ....

❑ ....

❑ ....

THINGS TO REMEMBER
(BECAUSE A BABY ATE MY BRAIN)

....

....

....

....

....

MEMORIES TO RECALL
(YEARS FROM NOW)

....

....

....

....

....

BABY NOTES
(WHAT YOU DID, LOVED, NEEDED)

....

....

....

....

....

....

....

....

....

....

....

....

....

WEANING NOTES
(WHAT YOU TRIED, LIKED, SPAT OUT)

....

....

....

....

....

....

....

....

....

....

....

....

....

Every mum
is DIFFERENT.
Every situation
is DIFFERENT.
Figure out what works
for YOUR family.

(and never take on board other people's
judgements or inadequacies.)

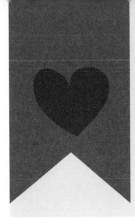

ON THIS DAY

DATE: _____

Spend time with other mums who inspire and boost you.

MY NOTES
(WHAT I LOVED, FELT, WISHED, NEEDED, STRUGGLED WITH, OVERCAME)

....

....

....

....

....

....

....

....

....

....

....

TO DO LIST

❏ ....

❏ ....

❏ ....

❏ ....

❏ ....

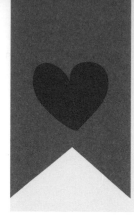

ON THIS DAY

DATE:

If anyone questions your decisions, maybe they're having trouble with their own.

MY NOTES
(WHAT I LOVED, FELT, WISHED, NEEDED, STRUGGLED WITH, OVERCAME)

....

....

....

....

....

....

....

....

....

....

....

TO DO LIST

❑ ....

❑ ....

❑ ....

❑ ....

❑ ....

THINGS TO REMEMBER
(BECAUSE A BABY ATE MY BRAIN)

....
....
....
....
....

MEMORIES TO RECALL
(YEARS FROM NOW)

....
....
....
....
....

BABY NOTES
(WHAT YOU DID, LOVED, NEEDED)

....
....
....
....
....
....
....
....
....
....
....
....
....
....

WEANING NOTES
(WHAT YOU TRIED, LIKED, SPAT OUT)

....
....
....
....
....
....
....
....
....
....
....
....
....
....

I'M ROCKING MY MUM MOJO.

AND THIS IS HOW:

....

....

....

....

....

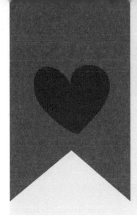

ON THIS DAY

DATE: _____

AMAZING.
AMAZING.
AMAZING.
That's you
by the way.

MY NOTES
(WHAT I LOVED, FELT, WISHED, NEEDED, STRUGGLED WITH, OVERCAME)

....

....

....

....

....

....

....

....

....

....

....

TO DO LIST

❑ ....

❑ ....

❑ ....

❑ ....

❑ ....

ON THIS DAY

DATE: _____

MY NOTES
(WHAT I LOVED, FELT, WISHED, NEEDED, STRUGGLED WITH, OVERCAME)

....

....

....

....

....

....

....

....

....

....

....

....

TO DO LIST

☐ ....

☐ ....

☐ ....

☐ ....

☐ ....

THINGS TO REMEMBER
(BECAUSE A BABY ATE MY BRAIN)

....

....

....

....

....

MEMORIES TO RECALL
(YEARS FROM NOW)

....

....

....

....

....

BABY NOTES
(WHAT YOU DID, LOVED, NEEDED)

....

....

....

....

....

....

....

....

....

....

....

....

....

WEANING NOTES
(WHAT YOU TRIED, LIKED, SPAT OUT)

....

....

....

....

....

....

....

....

....

....

....

....

....

THE END OF MATERNITY LEAVE

BYE BYE BABY BUBBLE

Coming to the end of the first year is an emotional time. Thinking about leaving the 'baby bubble' can be as scary as it was entering it, especially if it's coming earlier than you'd like because you're going back to work. You've undergone so many changes. Your baby's undergone so many changes. You've been joined at the hip, literally. It's very common to feel all sorts of nostalgia at this point in time, as you ponder how nearly a year has gone by so quickly (even though at times, the days have positively dragged).

GOING BACK TO WORK

Going back to work is different for everyone. For many mums, going back to work isn't a choice. It's a financial necessity and this can make it harder if, deep down, you'd prefer to be staying at home with your baby. Some mums, on the other hand, can't wait to get back to work and 'use their brains' again. Whatever your outlook, don't torment yourself with feelings of guilt. You've given your baby an amazing start in life and this is simply the next stage for you. Going back to work can be good for you both because children are stimulated by different influences and environments. As are you. There's no doubt that adding work into the motherhood mix means a lot of logistics, so be patient with yourself as you adjust to your new routine. Expect some upheaval at first and don't worry if your baby seems unsettled when you leave them. Babies have a habit of being hysterical in front of their parents and calming down the moment they've left. Take it day by day and, within as little as a week, you will both be well on your way and learning to make the most of the time you spend together.

GIVING UP WORK

If you've decided to give up work for the foreseeable future, there might be a niggle in the back of your mind. 'Am I doing the right thing? What if I lose all sense of who am I? Can I really do this day in, day out? Every. Single. Day?' It's very natural to have these thoughts. After all, your job has been a big part of your life. Establishing a daytime routine can really help you thrive in this stage of your life. Having a regular club/class or playgroup in the diary most days gives you a reason to go out and an opportunity to mix with other adults, something a lot of mums say they miss. You'll also find that as your baby starts to move, you'll need to work a bit harder to keep them amused. Open spaces and safe places are your friend and stop you from going insane when your newly toddling baby keeps getting everything out of your kitchen cupboards. For the tenth time that day. But being with a small person all the time can be draining, so always find time to do something that is just for you. Ask a friend or family member to take your baby to the park so you can have a couple of hours to yourself. You need this space to recharge. Never feel guilty for asking for it.

TAKE YOUR TIME

Whatever the next stage is for you, it's not going to be plain sailing. I've done every scenario possible whilst raising my three kids and I can tell you there's no perfect one when you're a mum. There will be days when juggling work and motherhood will send you over the edge and you'll wonder if it's worth all the effort. Likewise, when you've been at home with a meddling toddler all week, you might find yourself climbing the walls and questioning what you've done before reaching the catastrophic conclusion that you've ruined your life by giving up work. We all have days like this. We all survive them. Remind yourself why you're doing what you're doing right now. Whilst knowing that it doesn't have to be forever.

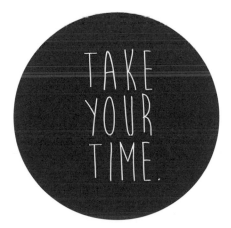

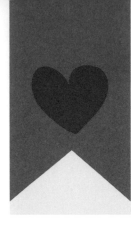

ON THIS DAY

DATE: _____

You will always be you, no matter what you do.

MY NOTES
(WHAT I LOVED, FELT, WISHED, NEEDED, STRUGGLED WITH, OVERCAME)

....

....

....

....

....

....

....

....

....

....

....

TO DO LIST

❑ ....

❑ ....

❑ ....

❑ ....

❑ ....

THINGS TO REMEMBER
(BECAUSE A BABY ATE MY BRAIN)

....
....
....
....
....

MEMORIES TO RECALL
(YEARS FROM NOW)

....
....
....
....
....

BABY NOTES
(WHAT YOU DID, LOVED, NEEDED)

....
....
....
....
....
....
....
....
....
....
....
....
....
....

WEANING NOTES
(WHAT YOU TRIED, LIKED, SPAT OUT)

....
....
....
....
....
....
....
....
....
....
....
....
....
....

Once you're a mother, there's no one path that's easier than another.

WALK YOUR OWN.

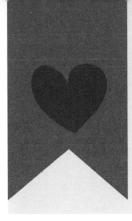

ON THIS DAY

DATE: _____

You rock.
Because you
have awesome
resources.

MY NOTES
(WHAT I LOVED, FELT, WISHED, NEEDED, STRUGGLED WITH, OVERCAME)

....

....

....

....

....

....

....

....

....

....

....

TO DO LIST

❑ ....

❑ ....

❑ ....

❑ ....

❑ ....

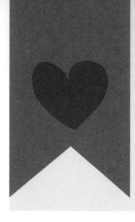

ON THIS DAY

DATE: _____

Every day you prove that you can do ANYTHING you put your mind to.

MY NOTES
(WHAT I LOVED, FELT, WISHED, NEEDED, STRUGGLED WITH, OVERCAME)

....

....

....

....

....

....

....

TO DO LIST

....

❏ ....

....

❏ ....

....

❏ ....

....

❏ ....

....

❏ ....

THINGS TO REMEMBER
(BECAUSE A BABY ATE MY BRAIN)

....
....
....
....
....

MEMORIES TO RECALL
(YEARS FROM NOW)

....
....
....
....
....

BABY NOTES
(WHAT YOU DID, LOVED, NEEDED)

....
....
....
....
....
....
....
....
....
....
....
....
....

WEANING NOTES
(WHAT YOU TRIED, LIKED, SPAT OUT)

....
....
....
....
....
....
....
....
....
....
....
....
....

TEN MONTHS!

THAT SURELY DESERVES:
A) CHOCOLATE
B) GIN
C) BOTH

THREE THINGS I FEEL GOOD ABOUT THIS MONTH:

1. ....

....

2. ....

....

3. ....

....

MONTH ELEVEN

This thing called motherhood.

IN IT FOR THE LONG-HAUL
(SOME THINGS TO REMEMBER)

MOTHERHOOD CHANGES YOU

You've already realised that when you become a mother, you throw your heart and soul into your kids. Literally. They steal your heart and they suck up your soul. And you will never be the same again. You are better in some ways. Less selfish. Patient to the point of passivity. And finally, you know REAL unconditional love. Because even when they're driving you absolutely bonkers, you'd still kill for them. In a heartbeat. In other ways you'll be worse. That unconditional love? Well, it can be a real sod when it comes to living your life independently of your kids, who will form the backdrop of every thought, plan and dream you ever have again.

TAKING TIME OUT

No one expects you to give yourself entirely to your child. And neither should you. But the reality is that, in the younger years at least, this is often exactly what happens. Alongside the other commitments in life, it can feel impossible to get any time for you. Unfortunately, the only way you'll actually ever get some is by taking it. Forcibly. Don't wait for it to just happen. Don't wait for someone to offer it to you. Don't feel guilty for needing it and asking for it. Schedule it in. Leave your child in the capable hands of someone else. And do something that makes you happy. You're showing your child that it's important to value yourself. That YOU are a person too. And that's a great lesson in self-esteem.

THERE WILL ALWAYS BE NEW CHALLENGES

Some days you will, of course, lose your cool. Completely and utterly. That's ok. As your baby grows into a toddler, you'll find yourself facing new challenges other than sleep deprivation. Because toddlers are completely different creatures to babies. They meddle. They tantrum. They learn the word, 'No!' You'll find that they want to do everything for themselves, without always having the skills to make this possible. You'll try to dress them. They'll scream, 'No!' You'll try to help them with a puzzle. They'll scream, 'No!' Once they can talk, every other sentence is, 'I do it'. So you'll wait. And you'll watch. As they put their leggings on their heads and force puzzle pieces together against their will. All the while losing precious minutes of your life that you'll never get back. Without ever reaching the end goal. You'll never really learn how to handle a toddler. Because their very nature defies all logic. All you can do is clap and wave them on like a deranged cheerleader. And accept that there is no right way to wear leggings. Because if you repress them now, you're just dragging out the pain. You will, however, learn what NOT to do with a toddler. You'll shop online for starters. And you won't turn your back for a second, unless you want to enjoy 'toilet roll soup' in the sink for lunch. Yup. These toddlers know how to party.

BEING THE MOTHER YOU WANT TO BE

The truth is that no one is ever the mother they imagined they'd be. Mainly because you can't really imagine motherhood until you've actually experienced it. The intensity and the relentlessness make it practically impossible to be the calm, ordered, perfect mother you had probably hoped to be. And as for being consistent all the time, there's no such thing. You can try and ensure your actions are consistent, sure (even this is hard some days). But your mood and temperament weren't consistent before becoming a mother so why should they be so now? In fact you're under more pressure than ever and the chances are you're going to be *more* temperamental, not less. So don't waste your time or energy feeling disappointed in your imperfect self. Ever. Motherhood's a marathon. Not a sprint. And you need to conserve your energy. The best thing about motherhood? You always get a second, third and millionth chance to do things differently. So always look forward. Because if you're not looking where you're going, you're going to trip over.

THERE IS NO BETTER MOTHER THAN YOU

You can never hear this enough. There is NO better mother for your child than YOU. But when the going gets tough, you're going to need to tell yourself this over and over again. Because human nature is such that you will always think otherwise. No one can soothe your child like you can. No one understands them like you do. THIS is your Supermum power. And THIS is what makes you your child's hero. Every single day.

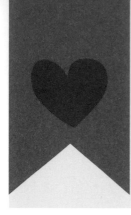

ON THIS DAY

DATE: _____

There are no mistakes in parenting. Just things you can learn from.

MY NOTES
(WHAT I LOVED, FELT, WISHED, NEEDED, STRUGGLED WITH, OVERCAME)

....

....

....

....

....

....

....

TO DO LIST

☐ ....

☐ ....

☐ ....

☐ ....

☐ ....

THINGS TO REMEMBER
(BECAUSE A BABY ATE MY BRAIN)

....
....
....
....
....

MEMORIES TO RECALL
(YEARS FROM NOW)

....
....
....
....
....

BABY NOTES
(WHAT YOU DID, LOVED, NEEDED)

....
....
....
....
....
....
....
....
....
....
....
....
....

WEANING NOTES
(WHAT YOU TRIED, LIKED, SPAT OUT)

....
....
....
....
....
....
....
....
....
....
....
....
....

Motherhood is about sacrifice.

(And eating biscuits. Also cake.)

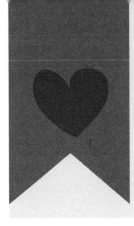

ON THIS DAY

DATE: _____

You are your child's hero. Even when you're feeling less than invincible.

MY NOTES
(WHAT I LOVED, FELT, WISHED, NEEDED, STRUGGLED WITH, OVERCAME)

....

....

....

....

....

....

....

TO DO LIST

☐ ....

....

☐ ....

....

☐ ....

....

☐ ....

....

☐ ....

....

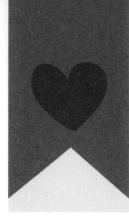

ON THIS DAY

DATE:
_____

Teach your child self-esteem by always valuing yourself.

MY NOTES
(WHAT I LOVED, FELT, WISHED, NEEDED, STRUGGLED WITH, OVERCAME)

....

....

....

....

....

....

....

....

....

....

....

TO DO LIST

❑ ....

❑ ....

❑ ....

❑ ....

❑ ....

THINGS TO REMEMBER
(BECAUSE A BABY ATE MY BRAIN)

....
....
....
....
....

MEMORIES TO RECALL
(YEARS FROM NOW)

....
....
....
....
....

BABY NOTES
(WHAT YOU DID, LOVED, NEEDED)

....
....
....
....
....
....
....
....
....
....
....
....
....

WEANING NOTES
(WHAT YOU TRIED, LIKED, SPAT OUT)

....
....
....
....
....
....
....
....
....
....
....
....
....

I promise to be kind to myself. ALWAYS.

BY REMEMBERING WHAT'S IMPORTANT TO ME:

1. ....
   ....

2. ....
   ....

3. ....
   ....

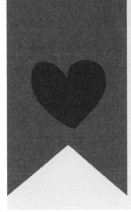

ON THIS DAY

DATE: _____

It's OK to lose your cool. So don't beat yourself up when you do.

MY NOTES
(WHAT I LOVED, FELT, WISHED, NEEDED, STRUGGLED WITH, OVERCAME)

....

....

....

....

....

....

....

....

....

....

....

TO DO LIST

☐ ....

☐ ....

☐ ....

☐ ....

☐ ....

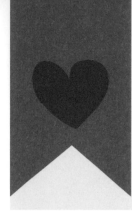

ON THIS DAY

DATE: _____

Shirk responsibility every now and then. And be the 'fun' parent.

MY NOTES
(WHAT I LOVED, FELT, WISHED, NEEDED, STRUGGLED WITH, OVERCAME)

....

....

....

....

....

....

....

....

....

....

....

TO DO LIST

❏ ....

❏ ....

❏ ....

❏ ....

❏ ....

THINGS TO REMEMBER
(BECAUSE A BABY ATE MY BRAIN)

....
....
....
....
....

MEMORIES TO RECALL
(YEARS FROM NOW)

....
....
....
....

BABY NOTES
(WHAT YOU DID, LOVED, NEEDED)

....
....
....
....
....
....
....
....
....
....
....
....
....

WEANING NOTES
(WHAT YOU TRIED, LIKED, SPAT OUT)

....
....
....
....
....
....
....
....
....
....
....
....
....

10 THINGS EVERY MOTHER LEARNS
(IN THE FIRST YEAR OF MOTHERHOOD)

1. **Getting a baby to sleep through the night is only half the story.** You are slowly learning that it's not over when the fat baby sleeps. What follows – your baby growing into a toddler with very firm ideas of their own – is harder, less predictable and more challenging than even Gina Ford tells you!

2. **You become an instant graduate in Advanced Multi-tasking.** Overnight, you've learned to wash, blow-dry and straighten your hair in 12 minutes. Whilst pouring a bowl of cereal and dressing your baby. You don't need one hour to do your hair as a relaxing solitary activity. And you don't miss this 'me time' at all. Not one little bit. Who are you kidding? The truth? You'll probably never straighten your hair again and will have bought a crate of dry shampoo instead.

3. **Patience can be learned and practiced.** As long as the following environmental factors are in place: eight hours sleep, wine and a full-time nanny.

4. **Motherhood can bring on involuntary swearing.** Mainly aimed at your strong-willed toddler. But can also be directed at complete strangers if they are doing any of the following things: chewing gum loudly, getting in your personal space or wasting your time (this list is not exhaustive).

5. **You will never again be able to control everything.** Most days you will struggle to control anything. Eventually, you admit defeat and give up even trying. This is called 'The End'.

6. **You will suddenly be able to explain your way out of any situation.** A skill born out of having to explain everything to a small, very intrusive person who has absolutely no regard for your privacy. This can be particularly useful when you're a) late for work b) late for a deadline c) late for anything. Just beware of any excuses which involve fairies or trolls. Adults usually see through these ones.

7. **You will not really do anything differently to your own parents.** You will try. You will think that you are. Then, one day, you'll hear your mother's voice and that really irritating phrase, 'I'm not telling you again'. And realise that the irritating voice is, in fact, yours.

8. **You will feel your child's sadness and pain as if it were your own.** Seeing your child feeling sad at the hands of someone else never gets easier to bear and, whilst this is completely natural, it is very dangerous if combined with a) lack of sleep b) hormones c) involuntary swearing.

9. **You will sometimes do the washing at 4.00AM.** This is called 'Using Your Time Effectively' or 'Finding The Only Slot In The Day When You Are On Your Own And Able To Do Anything Remotely Productive'.

10. **No one needs to go the toilet alone.** Since your baby's been crawling, you've learned that this is a fun team sport to be shared and enjoyed. Why poo alone when you can do it with an eager audience?

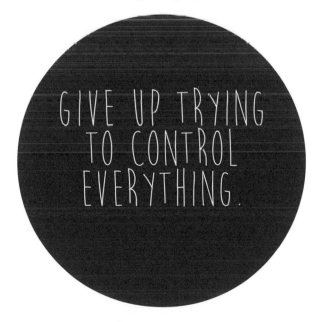

ON THIS DAY

DATE: _____

Don't be a martyr. Delegate. Ask for help. Accept help.

MY NOTES
(WHAT I LOVED, FELT, WISHED, NEEDED, STRUGGLED WITH, OVERCAME)

....

....

....

....

....

....

....

....

....

....

....

TO DO LIST

☐ ....

☐ ....

☐ ....

☐ ....

☐ ....

THINGS TO REMEMBER
(BECAUSE A BABY ATE MY BRAIN)

....

....

....

....

....

MEMORIES TO RECALL
(YEARS FROM NOW)

....

....

....

....

....

BABY NOTES
(WHAT YOU DID, LOVED, NEEDED)

....

....

....

....

....

....

....

....

....

....

....

....

WEANING NOTES
(WHAT YOU TRIED, LIKED, SPAT OUT)

....

....

....

....

....

....

....

....

....

....

....

....

Accept that everyone does things differently.

(there's no RIGHT way to make pasta and cheese.)

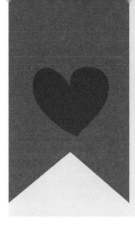

ON THIS DAY

DATE: _____

You're a mother.
Not a maid.
You can ask
for help with
household
chores.

MY NOTES
(WHAT I LOVED, FELT, WISHED, NEEDED, STRUGGLED WITH, OVERCAME)

....

....

....

....

....

....

....

....

....

....

TO DO LIST

❑ ....

❑ ....

❑ ....

❑ ....

❑ ....

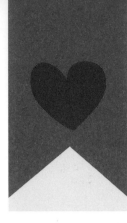

ON THIS DAY

DATE: _____

Behind every child is a brilliant mother. YOU.

MY NOTES
(WHAT I LOVED, FELT, WISHED, NEEDED, STRUGGLED WITH, OVERCAME)

....

....

....

....

....

....

....

TO DO LIST

❏ ....

❏ ....

❏ ....

❏ ....

❏ ....

THINGS TO REMEMBER
(BECAUSE A BABY ATE MY BRAIN)

....
....
....
....
....

MEMORIES TO RECALL
(YEARS FROM NOW)

....
....
....
....
....

BABY NOTES
(WHAT YOU DID, LOVED, NEEDED)

....
....
....
....
....
....
....
....
....
....
....
....

WEANING NOTES
(WHAT YOU TRIED, LIKED, SPAT OUT)

....
....
....
....
....
....
....
....
....
....
....
....

ELEVEN MONTHS!
YOU'VE DONE YOURSELF (AND YOUR BABY) PROUD.

THREE THINGS I ALWAYS WANT MY CHILD TO KNOW:

1. ....

....

2. ....

....

3. ....

....

MONTH TWELVE

Look how
far you've
come.

A CLOSING LETTER TO A NEW MUM

Dear New Mum,

So. A year ago, you were on the brink of becoming a mum. You were filled with expectation, apprehension and excitement. Do you remember that still? Twelve months on and you've achieved so much. You've got through some tough times and learned that you have more resilience and resourcefulness than you ever thought possible. You're probably feeling that motherhood has changed you in so many ways. But never forget that you are still YOU.

As your baby turns one, you might be filled with all manner of emotions. Joy and happiness, naturally. But perhaps also a little sadness that your baby isn't such a baby anymore. That this stage has passed. 'Did I make the most of it?' you may be wondering. 'What about the days I wished away?' But there's no need for regret. Because this isn't the end of your journey. It's the beginning of a new one. And in the same way you couldn't have ever imagined that feeling of having your newborn lie on you, you probably can't imagine that what comes next will be just as amazing. Yet, fortunately, it is.

Because watching your baby grow into a toddler is mesmerising. (It's also frustrating and challenging, but let's not focus on that right now.) It's not just the big milestones like seeing them learn to walk and talk, but also the smaller, subtler changes, like their personality gradually emerging. Or the first time they make you feel really proud because they do something loving or kind with an actual sense of self-awareness. Yes, your baby is becoming their own little person. And you've got the best seat in the house.

There will be challenges, of course there will. As your baby grows, so does your sense of responsibility. You'll worry about the consequences of any mistakes you perceive you're making. Are you damaging your child with every wrong turn you make? (You're not.) Is it your fault that your toddler is having a full on meltdown, in public? (It's not.) Please don't agonise over these things. So many aspects of a young child's behaviour are developmental phases. Like toddler tantrums, which are borne out of your child's frustration at not yet being able to communicate their needs effectively. In other words? You'll get through them. In their own, natural time. And then they'll be something else to baffle you. That's the nature of motherhood.

You'll need to be made of strong stuff some days. But you've already shown yourself you're more than capable of that. Sometimes, you'll find yourself at the mercy of others. Because whilst most people are pretty accommodating of babies (they're generally cute to look at), a tantruming toddler or stroppy three-year-old doesn't always get quite the same reception. People unrealistically expect them to know better and, in the process, you may become privy to unwanted opinions. Strangers' opinions, even. It can be incredibly upsetting when you feel like you're being judged. Especially, when you're not feeling confident in what you're doing anyway. Sadly, we've all been there. Building up a resilience to this sort of behaviour comes with experience and, often, with having more children. In the meantime, try to detach yourself if someone criticises your parenting. 'What do they know?' ask yourself. 'They're watching one tiny snapshot of our lives. They don't know anything.' Always believe in yourself. Not in someone else's version of you.

Finally, always believe in your child. Because, believe me, there will be times when you don't. When someone else's insensitivity or arrogance causes you to compare them to another child who might be better behaved or more confident or whatever it is that you feel your own child struggles with. But every child is unique and every child learns in their own time. So never let someone fool you into pitting your child against theirs.

You and your child are wonderful and EXACTLY the way you are meant to be.

Amy x

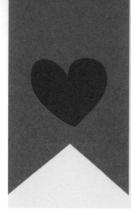

ON THIS DAY

DATE: _____

Motherhood will always pose challenges. And you'll always work through them.

MY NOTES
(WHAT I LOVED, FELT, WISHED, NEEDED, STRUGGLED WITH, OVERCAME)

....

....

....

....

....

....

....

....

....

....

....

TO DO LIST

☐ ....

☐ ....

☐ ....

☐ ....

☐ ....

THINGS TO REMEMBER
(BECAUSE A BABY ATE MY BRAIN)

....
....
....
....
....

MEMORIES TO RECALL
(YEARS FROM NOW)

....
....
....
....
....

BABY NOTES
(WHAT YOU DID, LOVED, NEEDED)

....
....
....
....
....
....
....
....
....
....
....
....
....

WEANING NOTES
(WHAT YOU TRIED, LIKED, SPAT OUT)

....
....
....
....
....
....
....
....
....
....
....
....
....

THE MOTHERHOOD MANTRA

1. No guilt
2. Things pass
3. You are enough

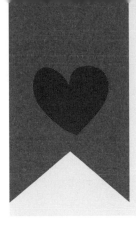

ON THIS DAY

DATE: _____

Don't allow yourself to get lost. Spend some time with YOU.

MY NOTES
(WHAT I LOVED, FELT, WISHED, NEEDED, STRUGGLED WITH, OVERCAME)

....

....

....

....

....

....

....

....

....

....

....

TO DO LIST

❑ ....

❑ ....

❑ ....

❑ ....

❑ ....

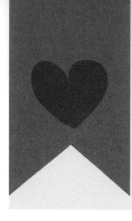

ON THIS DAY

DATE: _____

Remember when you thought you couldn't do it? And then you did?

MY NOTES
(WHAT I LOVED, FELT, WISHED, NEEDED, STRUGGLED WITH, OVERCAME)

....

....

....

....

....

....

....

....

....

....

....

TO DO LIST

☐ ....

☐ ....

☐ ....

☐ ....

☐ ....

THINGS TO REMEMBER
(BECAUSE A BABY ATE MY BRAIN)

....

....

....

....

....

MEMORIES TO RECALL
(YEARS FROM NOW)

....

....

....

....

....

BABY NOTES
(WHAT YOU DID, LOVED, NEEDED)

....

....

....

....

....

....

....

....

....

....

....

....

....

WEANING NOTES
(WHAT YOU TRIED, LIKED, SPAT OUT)

....

....

....

....

....

....

....

....

....

....

....

....

....

THE SCHOOL OF MOTHERHOOD

AWARDS

·····································

DISTINCTION

★

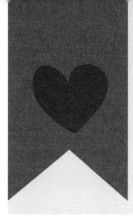

ON THIS DAY

DATE: _____

Have a flexible approach to parenting. Try not to worry about every little thing.

MY NOTES
(WHAT I LOVED, FELT, WISHED, NEEDED, STRUGGLED WITH, OVERCAME)

....
....
....
....
....
....
....

....

....

....

....

....

TO DO LIST

❑ ....

❑ ....

❑ ....

❑ ....

❑ ....

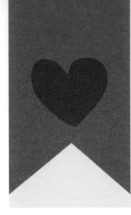

ON THIS DAY

DATE: _____

Whenever you find yourself struggling, remember how far you've come.

MY NOTES
(WHAT I LOVED, FELT, WISHED, NEEDED, STRUGGLED WITH, OVERCAME)

....

....

....

....

....

....

....

TO DO LIST

- ☐ ....
- ☐ ....
- ☐ ....
- ☐ ....
- ☐ ....

....

....

....

....

THINGS TO REMEMBER
(BECAUSE A BABY ATE MY BRAIN)

....

....

....

....

....

MEMORIES TO RECALL
(YEARS FROM NOW)

....

....

....

....

....

BABY NOTES
(WHAT YOU DID, LOVED, NEEDED)

....

....

....

....

....

....

....

....

....

....

....

....

....

WEANING NOTES
(WHAT YOU TRIED, LIKED, SPAT OUT)

....

....

....

....

....

....

....

....

....

....

....

....

....

LIVE MOTHERHOOD YOUR WAY

Put your hands up if you're tired. **Really tired.** Tired of not having enough headspace. Tired of all the demands on your time. Tired of **small people** calling your name. And not even the name you were given. But some generic term called **'Mummeeee'.** Are you fed up with doing it all at home? Being the strong one? Being perfect? Being **selfless.** Do you have an overwhelming desire to escape some days? Pack a bag, grab your **passport** and get on a flight back to your 20s. On an all-inclusive package that includes freedom, sanity and wild nights followed by lazy mornings. And a shed load of **cocktails.** Well guess what, you can. It's in your power, mostly. Not escaping literally. But mentally. You see, in many ways we've made it this way. Our desire for equality. For **perfection.** To have it all when we know we can't. It's our tendency to be overbearing and controlling. Our insistence that if we want it done right, we must do it ourselves. A tendency that multiplies when we bear children and we've got even more on our plates. It's our bizarre choice to live like this. In **motherhood martyrdom**. Our edges harden. We forget how to show vulnerability. Even though we still feel it. We lose the ability to finish sentences and conversations. And we communicate less with our partners and **pray** instead that they'll **read our minds.** But they aren't mind-readers. Never have been. Never will be. So we become resentful. And the edges harden more. We're exhausted from doing it for ourselves. We miss **chivalry.** More than anything, we want a **bloody good lie-in.** So let's change what we can. Ourselves. Remember what you like about yourself. **Give up** the need to be everything to everyone. It's impossible and it's unfulfilling. Take a step back and accept **you can't have everything.** No one does. Then look at what you really want and ask for it. If you don't ask, you don't get. It's that simple. Tell your partner you **love** them instead of gritting your teeth. **Smile** when you feel like frowning. Delegate. **Share responsibility.** Even if this means installing a big neon sign pointing to the washing machine. And **accept** that everyone does things differently. There is no right way to make pasta and cheese. **Shirk responsibility** every now and again. It will do you good and remind you how many of the demands on your **time** come only from you. **Make time for yourself.** Because time won't make room for you. And this is it. Right now. **YOUR LIFE.** So live it wisely. Live it happily. **LIVE IT YOUR WAY.**

SURVIVING THE FIRST BIRTHDAY

1. **Don't have a massive party.** You'll spend the whole time organising stuff and forget to take stock of the day itself and your baby. Keep it simple. A few people you love. And a bowl of cheese savouries. Do that once and no one will want to come to your parties again anyway. Job done.

2. **Don't make a speech after drinking gin.** It will make you want to share every vivid emotion that's running through your veins.

3. **Don't worry if your baby sleeps through the entire party.** In time you'll see that this is a good thing and means that *you* can enjoy yourself. Which is the whole point anyway, right?

4. **Let your baby taste the nectar.** Woo hoo! Your baby can eat honey AND drink cow's milk. Talk about coming of age. (Talk about an anti-climax.)

5. **Don't give your baby too much cake.** If, until now, your baby has existed on a diet of organic carrots, don't give them a whole slab of cake 'because it's their birthday'. Unless you want to be scraping sick off their sheets at around 10.00PM. Wean them onto their sugar addiction gradually. Soon, it's all they'll want to eat.

6. **Stop counting your baby in weeks.** If you haven't already done this, the first birthday is definitely the time to stop. 'My baby is 53 weeks' makes you sound a bit, erm, crackers.

7. **Take nostalgia for what it is.** You'll probably be thinking sentimental things like, 'Awww, my baby isn't a baby anymore,' leading to crazy thoughts like, 'Perhaps we should have another one?'. NOOOOOOOO! This is what Mother Nature wants you to do. Have you forgotten the hideous, sleepless nights? Pour yourself another gin and stop it. Right now.

8. **Congratulate yourself.** You made it. You, who couldn't keep a pot plant alive, have nurtured a human being to their first birthday! You've done yourself and your baby proud.

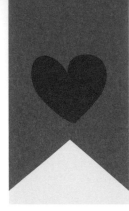

ON THIS DAY

DATE: _____

Never let anyone steal your mum mojo by undermining you.

MY NOTES
(WHAT I LOVED, FELT, WISHED, NEEDED, STRUGGLED WITH, OVERCAME)

....

....

....

....

....

....

....

....

....

....

....

TO DO LIST

❏ ....

❏ ....

❏ ....

❏ ....

❏ ....

THINGS TO REMEMBER
(BECAUSE A BABY ATE MY BRAIN)

....

....

....

....

....

MEMORIES TO RECALL
(YEARS FROM NOW)

....

....

....

....

....

BABY NOTES
(WHAT YOU DID, LOVED, NEEDED)

....

....

....

....

....

....

....

....

....

....

....

....

....

WEANING NOTES
(WHAT YOU TRIED, LIKED, SPAT OUT)

....

....

....

....

....

....

....

....

....

....

....

....

....

BELIEVE IN
YOURSELF.

(look at the journey
you've been on.)

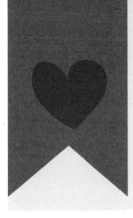

ON THIS DAY

DATE: _____

Your baby's where they are today. Because of YOU.

MY NOTES
(WHAT I LOVED, FELT, WISHED, NEEDED, STRUGGLED WITH, OVERCAME)

....

....

....

....

....

....

....

....

....

....

TO DO LIST

☐ ....

☐ ....

☐ ....

☐ ....

☐ ....

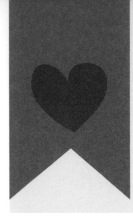

ON THIS DAY

There's nothing you can't do. Only things you have yet to do.

DATE: _____

MY NOTES
(WHAT I LOVED, FELT, WISHED, NEEDED, STRUGGLED WITH, OVERCAME)

....

....

....

....

....

....

....

....

....

....

....

TO DO LIST

- ☐ ....
- ☐ ....
- ☐ ....
- ☐ ....
- ☐ ....

THINGS TO REMEMBER
(BECAUSE A BABY ATE MY BRAIN)

....
....
....
....
....

MEMORIES TO RECALL
(YEARS FROM NOW)

....
....
....
....
....

BABY NOTES
(WHAT YOU DID, LOVED, NEEDED)

....
....
....
....
....
....
....
....
....
....
....
....
....
....

WEANING NOTES
(WHAT YOU TRIED, LIKED, SPAT OUT)

....
....
....
....
....
....
....
....
....
....
....
....
....
....

ONE YEAR!
YOU DID IT!

MY THREE DEFINING MOMENTS THIS YEAR:

1. ....
   ....

2. ....
   ....

3. ....
   ....

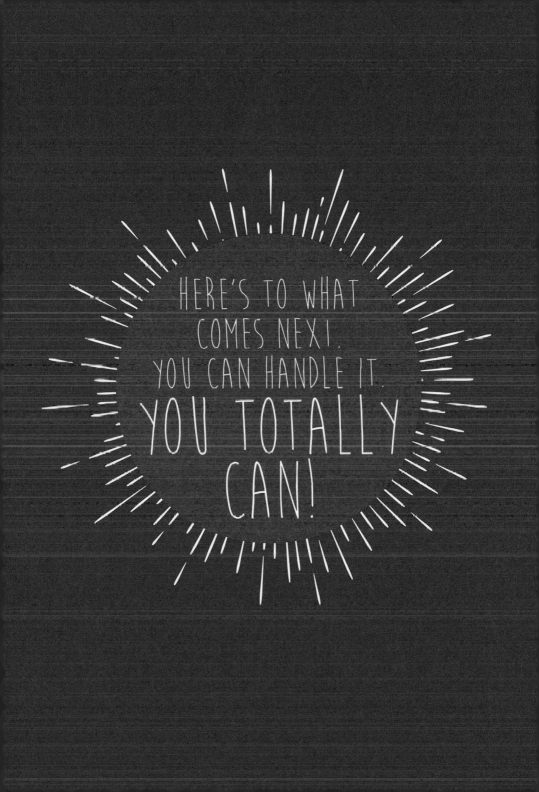

MILESTONE CHARTS

I wish I could remember when my baby...

Use the list below as inspiration to record your
baby's milestones. Because you WILL forget.
(There's a few for you too.)

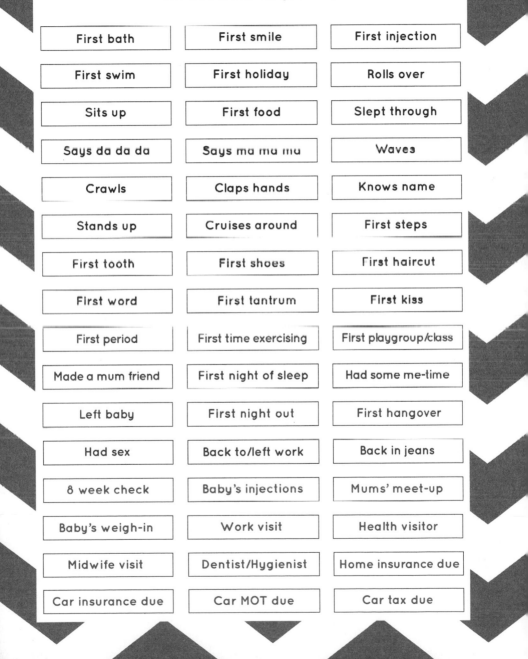

First bath	First smile	First injection
First swim	First holiday	Rolls over
Sits up	First food	Slept through
Says da da da	Says ma ma ma	Waves
Crawls	Claps hands	Knows name
Stands up	Cruises around	First steps
First tooth	First shoes	First haircut
First word	First tantrum	First kiss
First period	First time exercising	First playgroup/class
Made a mum friend	First night of sleep	Had some me-time
Left baby	First night out	First hangover
Had sex	Back to/left work	Back in jeans
8 week check	Baby's injections	Mums' meet-up
Baby's weigh-in	Work visit	Health visitor
Midwife visit	Dentist/Hygienist	Home insurance due
Car insurance due	Car MOT due	Car tax due

Month One

1	17
2	18
3	19
4	20
5	21
6	22
7	23
8	24
9	25
10	26
11	27
12	28
13	29
14	30
15	31
16	

Month Two

1	17
2	18
3	19
4	20
5	21
6	22
7	23
8	24
9	25
10	26
11	27
12	28
13	29
14	30
15	31
16	

Month Three

1	17
2	18
3	19
4	20
5	21
6	22
7	23
8	24
9	25
10	26
11	27
12	28
13	29
14	30
15	31
16	

Month Four

1	17
2	18
3	19
4	20
5	21
6	22
7	23
8	24
9	25
10	26
11	27
12	28
13	29
14	30
15	31
16	

Month Five

1	17
2	18
3	19
4	20
5	21
6	22
7	23
8	24
9	25
10	26
11	27
12	28
13	29
14	30
15	31
16	

Month Six

1	17
2	18
3	19
4	20
5	21
6	22
7	23
8	24
9	25
10	26
11	27
12	28
13	29
14	30
15	31
16	

Month Seven

1	17
2	18
3	19
4	20
5	21
6	22
7	23
8	24
9	25
10	26
11	27
12	28
13	29
14	30
15	31
16	

Month Eight

1	17
2	18
3	19
4	20
5	21
6	22
7	23
8	24
9	25
10	26
11	27
12	28
13	29
14	30
15	31
16	

Month Nine

1	17
2	18
3	19
4	20
5	21
6	22
7	23
8	24
9	25
10	26
11	27
12	28
13	29
14	30
15	31
16	

Month Ten

1	17
2	18
3	19
4	20
5	21
6	22
7	23
8	24
9	25
10	26
11	27
12	28
13	29
14	30
15	31
16	

Month Eleven

1	17
2	18
3	19
4	20
5	21
6	22
7	23
8	24
9	25
10	26
11	27
12	28
13	29
14	30
15	31
16	

Month Twelve

1		17	
2		18	
3		19	
4		20	
5		21	
6		22	
7		23	
8		24	
9		25	
10		26	
11		27	
12		28	
13		29	
14		30	
15		31	
16			

NOTES

NOTES

NOTES

NOTES

NOTES

NOTES

NOTES

NOTES

NOTES

NOTES

NOTES

ACKNOWLEDGEMENTS

The more time that passes, the more I feel as though *The New Mum's Notebook* created itself. But of course it didn't. It is a collaboration of minds.

First and foremost I must thank Gina. She patiently designed every beautiful page. Our firstborns went to nursery and now go to school together. When I asked her in the playground if she fancied doing it, it was going to be less than 200 pages. Then it grew. And grew. We sat around my kitchen table every week choosing patterns and laying it out. There isn't anyone else who could have done what she did.

Next, my gorgeous friend Luce: a talented and savvy interiors stylist, my NCT friend and someone I am happy to see every day at the school gates. She is the person I go to because I know I will ALWAYS get an honest and intelligent answer from her. When I ran the *Notebook* past her, she simply said, 'Yes'. When we saw the first finished copy she said, 'This is beautiful. Someone is going to take this off your hands, trust me.' Seven months later I got the offer from Hutchinson at Penguin Random House. She styled the beautiful photography and has been there all the way. As has Gareth, Luce's other half, who designed my ecommerce website and swiftly came on board as marketing guru. Hugely talented, but also patient and insightful, he would reassure me (quoting Ronan Keating's 'Life is a Roller Coaster') when I wondered if self-publishing thousands of copies of a hardback book and storing them at home was a bit bonkers. To Max, who shot the beautiful photography, what a brilliant and fun day we had! To my beautiful NCT friend, fellow PA and mum of three, Jastine, for proofing the book and her continual encouragement in all that I do. To my friend, Tom, who shifted all 3000 books into my house on the hottest day of the year whilst I sat on a beach drinking pina coladas (sorry).

To all the wonderful and supportive friends motherhood has brought me: my quirky NCT girls; my lovely school mums; my hilarious playgroup mums; my Instagram and Facebook friends – you always lift me and remind me that we're never alone.

Thank you to everyone who follows my blog, has bought a copy of the *Notebook*, shared it and told me how much it means to them. To all the lovely stockists who took a chance on an independent author and sell the *Notebook* with such enthusiasm, working with you has seen one of the most enjoyable parts of this venture. To my lovely, warm agent, Laura, who I liked from the minute we met, for believing in me and the *Notebook*, taking it to the next level and being part of the dream team that I know I have. To Sarah, my publisher, and the rest of the team at Hutchinson, thank you for saying the LOVELIEST things about the *Notebook* and writing an offer letter so enthusiastic and warm that I pretty much texted it to everyone I know. I am so grateful to have your expertise and brilliance.

To my parents, who have always let me do my own (often crazy) thing and instilled in me the belief that a good work ethic will eventually see you through. Thank you for always being there and for being proud of me. To my sister, a kindred spirit, no words needed except to say that I hope my girls one day have what we have.

Finally, to my three wonderfully individual, and often eccentric, kids. This notebook would never have happened without you! It took YOU to fulfil my dream of becoming a published writer. You fill my life with joy, chaos and noise. I want you to always believe. Because marvellous things happen when you do.

Amy x